Cupping Therapy

How to Effectively Use Cupping Therapy in
Healing

*(The Definitive Guide on How to Effectively
Use Cupping Therapy)*

Dwayne Kepner

Published By **Jackson Denver**

Dwayne Kepner

Cupping Therapy: How to Effectively Use Cupping Therapy in Healing (The Definitive Guide on How to Effectively Use Cupping Therapy)

ISBN 978-1-77485-462-4

Legal & Disclaimer

The information contained in this book is not designed to replace or take the place of any form of medicine or professional medical advice. The information in this book has been provided for educational and entertainment purposes only.

The information contained in this book has been compiled from sources deemed reliable, and it is accurate to the best of the Author's knowledge; however, the Author cannot guarantee its accuracy and validity and cannot be held liable for any errors or omissions. Changes are periodically made to this book. You must consult your doctor or get professional medical advice before using any of the suggested remedies, techniques, or information in this book.

Upon using the information contained in this book, you agree to hold harmless the Author from and against any damages, costs, and expenses, including any legal fees potentially resulting from the application of any of the information provided by this guide. This disclaimer applies to any damages or injury caused by the use and application, whether directly or indirectly, of any advice or information presented, whether for breach of contract, tort, negligence, personal injury, criminal intent, or under any other cause of action.

You agree to accept all risks of using the information presented inside this book. You need to consult a professional medical practitioner in order to ensure you are both able and healthy enough to participate in this program.

TABLE OF CONTENTS

Introduction

Cupping therapy is an old method of medical treatment that is commonly used in lieu of medical treatment. The method involves placing cups over the skin of the patient for a short time to create a process known as suction takes place. This procedure offers a wide variety of benefits that include relief from discomfort, inflammation and the sensation of relaxation, increased flow of blood and the overall health of the patient. Cupping therapy is also a method by which it is possible to get a deep massage of the tissues. The cups for therapeutic use employed for this procedure are typically made from glass, bamboo as well as silicone and Earthenware.

It is not a surprise that nowadays, cupping therapy is rapidly becoming well-known, despite the fact that it's an traditional practice that is dated back to the ancient Egyptian, Middle Eastern and Chinese civilizations. The evidence of its longevity is found in the medical journal known as Ebers Papyrus where a description of how in 1.550 B.C it was that the Egyptians employed cupping therapies is provided. In addition, because those from the West are still experimenting with this method, Chinese have been using it since the year 1000 B.C. Numerous studies have proven that this technique is used in numerous variations, which means that it could be utilized differently from one culture to the next. It's also possible that this method is older than we think.

Another point that should be noted this is the fact that cupping therapy provides numerous advantages that are greater than ones derived from modern medical practices. One of the most significant advantages of this method, whether to treat or cure is that, unlike other treatments Cupping is not associated with negative side effects that are in opposition to pharmaceutical medications. That is to say there is nothing to lose using this method as an alternative treatment method. In reality, a number of studies have demonstrated that this technique aids in increasing the immunity of a person and, consequently accelerates his recovery , without the requirement to take additional forms of medication.

It is well-known that in most cultures across the world, making resolutions at the start of the year is an established custom. In the hope of sustaining well-being throughout the year is usually among the top priorities on people's New Year's resolutions. In this regard, a lot of people choose to use cupping treatments while also attempting to enjoy the benefits of an ancient Chinese custom and, while doing so benefit from a variety of health benefits all through the year. The practice of cupping is described as a type of inversed massage instead of applying pressure to muscles, cups utilized to facilitate suction. These cups is in turn the suctions that generate enough force to push the skin muscles, and tissues upwards.

These days, a lot of people are combining cupping therapies with other treatments like acupuncture, to aid their health and prevent certain illnesses although cupping therapy doesn't have to be paired with other therapies to produce excellent outcomes. The long-term results are mostly because of the chain of reactions that occur immediately following the suction treatment on the tissues, muscles, and the skin. This then leads to the vacuum effect, which improves blood circulation, reduces down body temperatures , and aids in detoxifying the body in the

3

process. In normal circumstances, when applying the technique there is a tightening feeling experienced on the body in which the cup is set. The sensation is usually called a feeling of relaxation as a result of it has calming effects.

Based on the comfort level of the patient as well as the evaluation performed by the therapist or the medical professional during the session, the cup can be moved around or remain in its place. It also decides on the length of time that the cups should be placed upon the body. It is important to note that cupping therapy differs based on the patient's condition or pain on a specific day. While the most commonly used location where cups can be placed for a treatment is on the lower back it's not the only area in the human body which could be utilized. Therapists typically choose the most fleshy areas of the body to achieve better results.

When cupping, the area where the cups were placed can change in the form of blue, red or purple. This is usually the case in the event of an injury or the forceful pressure placed on the cupping area. It is a sign that skin discolorations can be seen on the skin for a couple of days or weeks. The good thing is that it's pain completely painless. After the skin discolorations have gone, the treatment is able to be repeated until the skin condition is completely cured.

Michael Phelps and Natalie Coughlin cupping Olympians...

Certain Olympians have been using cupping therapy in the present. This is evident from the purple circular bruises on their bodies. This is why they caused a lot of questions to be addressed by the general public. Michael Phelps is one of the numerous Olympic swimmers who use cupping therapy. As he stated in 2015 the need to boost the amount of time he worked out and also intensify his swimming to prepare for Rio. The result was that he began using cupping to help relax muscles and speedy recovery aiding him in achieving his goals and priorities.

According to Phelps Cupping therapy, according to Phelps, is not a cure per se however it aids in keeping his fascia well-lubricated. This lets his muscles move with greater ease. This is due to the fact that, unlike regular massages, which push muscles and fascia downwards cupping is a method of pulling the fascia and muscle layers apart just like the separating of layers of pastry flake. This facilitates the flow of blood and fluids throughout the body and keeps them hydrated and assisting to move more easily. Michael Phelps confirms that he has at minimum two cups every week, even though it can leave marks on his body.

Natalie Coughlin, the former team USA swimmer, has introduced Michael Phelps to cupping therapy. According Coughlin the red marks left behind after treatment are a badge of honour and serve as evidence of muscles that have become sore following an intense workout. Coughlin was first introduced to this treatment when she was a part of an Australian swimmers. She believes that cupping therapy played a crucial role in speeding her recovery and the recovery of her team members which has allowed them to be competitive night and day without interruptions.

The aim for this book is to provide some understanding not only of how cupping therapy works but also the benefits it brings to Olympic athletes and the diverse ways in which this method is able to heal the body naturally. In this book, you'll discover how to use this method in the comfort at home, and experience the benefits associated with its use.

Chapter 1: Sports Cupping 101: What You Should Be Aware Of The Latest Sports Trend

A muscle is similar to the elastic bands. It stretches and moves. The fascia is the layer that covers the muscles. If the muscle is connected by the fascia it is not able to extend or move. This may limit the movement of the muscle and could impact athletic performance.

Cupping therapy removes the adhesions between muscles and fascia to improve the performance of your biomechanics. It also allows you to move more freely and enhance you physical efficiency.

Cupping therapy is a method which involves a skilled therapist placing an earthenware, glass or bamboo cup over the skin in order to create suction. This suction improves blood flow, and reduces inflammation and pain.

Cupping is the most effective treatment used by famous athletes such as Michael Phelps. Wang Qun, a celebrated Chinese swimmer proudly displayed her cupping marks at the 2008 Olympics that took place in Beijing. The athletes who are part of the New York Mets are also employing cupping therapy to enhance their performance. Cupping therapy is not just employed by athletes. Many other famous people make use of cupping to improve their health . Some of them include Jennifer Aniston, Gwyneth Paltrow, Maria Menounos, Victoria Beckham, David Arquette, and Jessica Simpson.

For those who don't realize that cupping therapy isn't something new. Actually, it's been around for more than 2000 years.

The history of Cupping

In terms of the past Cupping was a practice which was used in various areas of the world, like Asia, Africa and Europe. In the early days, many worried about the existence of evil spirits as well as the potential for these spirits inflicting illness. African medicine men would make hollows from animal horns, then hollow them out, and then cut off the ends. They used this to create an unorthodox yet effective method of cupping. By using their mouths and tongue, they created suction in the animal horns to treat snake bites, boils or skin lesions. To ensure suction they chewed on leaves mixed with saliva to close holes in the animal horn.

Cupping records written down are from in the 2nd century BC. Cupping was recorded in a book written by Bo Shu, written on silk, and was written in the Han Dynasty. Cupping for its therapeutic benefits was first introduced in a book that was written by Zouhou Fang in the year 28 AD.

Cupping is widely used and documented in China. In the early 500s the first Chinese surgeon employed this technique during surgery to help to keep blood from the site of surgery. Through time the procedure was adapted from simple horns, into bamboos, clay, and glass cups.

The practice of Cupping Therapy also became very popular in Egypt in the past. In fact, it was mentioned in an antiquated Egyptian text known as The Ebers Papyrus. It is among the oldest textbooks on medicine. Cupping was popularized within Ancient Greece. Hippocrates the father medical science, employed cupping to treat structural issues as well as internal ailments. It was believed by Hippocrates that cupping could be used to treat the majority of diseases. A number of Greek doctors relied on cupping to improve the alignment of the spine in patients.

Cupping eventually became popular across many countries of Europe along with South as well as North America. Cupping was widely utilized by American as well as European physicians in the early part in the 1800s. It was employed in private and hospital practices. At this point a method known as wet cupping, also known as Hijama was becoming more well-known throughout the Middle East. It's a method which involves the therapist making small cuts in the skin of the patient to drain blood, toxins as well as poisons, out.

In the second quarter in the 1800s the demand for cupping treatment declined because of the development of a brand new medical model.

In the 1950s, China came together along with Soviet Union. Soviet Union to conduct an extensive study on cupping technique. This study confirmed that the effectiveness of cupping. Cupping has been extensively used in hospitals owned by the government in China.

Cupping came back in the West as a popular trend after Gwyneth Paltrow proudly displayed her cupping marks at New York Film Festival. Since then, numerous other celebrities like Jennifer Aniston, Justin Bieber, Kim Kardashian, and Victoria Beckham followed suit. The trend was adopted by sports celebrities like Serena Williams.

The cupping treatment became more popular after swimming superstars were seen sporting cupping marks at the 2016 Rio Olympics. Famous Olympian Michael Phelps was also photographed using the cupping technique for muscle healing during the Under Armour ad.

Cupping in sports is currently rising as a trend in the sport of sports. Actually, it's advised by numerous physical therapists and sports coaches. It is mostly used to aid in the recovery of muscles.

Cupping along with the Qi

Before we look at the process of cupping therapy, we should first consider the concept of Qi. Qi is the main concept used in Traditional Chinese Medicine techniques such as cupping and acupuncture.

Qi refers to the bioelectric energy that is present in each human being. It is identical to the concept of prana found in the ancient Indian medicine. This is the source of energy which defends the body from pathogens external to it like the pollution, bacteria, weather and viruses. It also helps to cool and warm the body whenever required. Qi flows through energy points within the body, referred to as meridians, to stimulate growth and avoid stagnation. If you're able to maintain a healthy Qi, you'll be active and be able to maintain your endurance. This boosts your sporting performance.

Being able to balance your qi improves your ability to concentrate and enhances your overall health and wellbeing. If your chi flows easily and opposing energies of your body,"yin and Yang" are balanced and balanced, you'll be successful throughout your life: your career, health and relationships, as well as personal growth.

If your Qi isn't flowing properly within the body's tissues, then you'll feel fatigue, as well as other health problems. This can cause anxiety and depression. This can adversely affect the performance of your sport. Qi imbalance can cause infertility as well as allergies, liver diseases and memory loss, as well as illnesses of the immune system, and severe medical conditions. It can affect the functioning of your digestive system, liver the brain, lymphatic system as well as the cardiovascular system and reproductive organs.

There are many elements that hinder the flow of chi throughout your body, for example, anxiety, stress, inadequate of exercise, or a poor diet. Training too much can lead to stagnation of qi.

Cupping therapy helps to ease stagnation and clears your qi through increasing the circulation of blood in your body. It is a method to boost the body's natural energy flow. It also activates and increases the body's self-healing abilities.

Cupping in Sports

Cupping is a relatively new yet effective method of rehabilitation training. It assists in stimulating the fascia by applying negative pressure which pushes the skin to the outside, this is in contrast to the way massage is typically done. When massage is performed, pressure is applied to the skin in order to reach the muscles below. When cupping, the suction assists in moving stagnant blood, as well as loosening muscle and fascia which are tight.

Sports injuries are extremely frequent. This is particularly true for contact sports like football, hockey and rugby. The body is subject to a number of procedures to heal itself naturally.

The phases of Healing

The initial stages of healing are triggered by the healing of an injury. In this crucial moment the body goes through hemostasis. Platelets will move toward the location of injury and release substances like cytokines, chemicals, as well as hormones.

The blood vessels that line the area narrow, reducing the flow of blood towards the site of injury. The skin that is exposed on the site of injury will trigger the process of platelet aggregation, which aids in helping the platelets form a clump, forming an obstruction and stop bleeding. When the platelets clump together on collagen, this causes the platelets to release chemical (coagulation cascades) which trigger the initial phase of healing of the wound.

1. INFLAMMATORY PhASE

The formation of clots stops. The initial vasoconstriction response will cease around 10 minutes following the injury. Then, it is followed by a longer time of vasodilation. Vasodilation increases blood flow within the region and also histamines, prostaglandins and kinins as well as leukotrienes. The damaged cells are then destroyed and macrophages wash off all particles and bacteria that have accumulated caused by the injury. This causes changes to the pH of the skin that can cause discomfort. Macrophages play an important part in the whole process because they release a variety of chemicals that help in the process of tissue growth.

2. PROLIFERATION PHASE

This is the stage where new tissues and cells form. It happens in different stages.

Epithelization is the time when the wound is closed slowly over with the help of cell migration to the area of injury. It creates a separation between the injury and the surrounding environment.

Fibroplasia can be seen around 3-5 days after the injury. It can last between 14 and 15 days before it is finished. Fibroblast are responsible for creating collagen glycosaminoglycans, fibronectin, elastin and proteases. The inflammation subsides, and collagen starts connecting the cells.

Angiogenesis Blood flow is crucial to ensure the health and growth of cells that are being created. The blood vessels that are created during this stage. made in this phase when it is needed. However, blood vessels that are not needed are eliminated via apoptosis.

Contraction - This is the stage in which the edges of the wound are moved toward the center, in an attempt to close the top and join those newly created cells.

3. MATURATION PHASE

In this stage the wound goes through the last phases of healing. Collagen remains created and eliminated when not necessary. The wound continues to heal but the skin that is grafted in is not as strong in comparison to the non-injured region. It may take up to 21 days following the injury before collagen begins to stabilize.

When is sports cupping not contraindicated?

Cupping during sports injuries is not recommended in the ACUTE phase. It is typically in the initial 48-hour period following the injury. It is associated by an increase in blood flow around the injured area and swelling. If there is evidence for bleeding (whether internal or external) or inflammation, as well as fractures, open wounds, and ruptures of the tendon completely Cupping shouldn't be done. Skin injuries aren't the only ones that require cupping as it's usually associated with open wounds.

What is the best time to start cupping sports?

Cupping for sports is performed in the recovery phase which is the period that physical therapy is suggested. It is believed to be efficient when used to assist in muscle recovery and to improve blood flow to the region.

It is crucial to note that for the healing and recovery of muscles oxygenation and blood flow are crucial elements. Both of these can be improved and increased through cupping therapy.

The way the Cupping Works

Cupping therapy is where an therapist places the skin using a glass to create suction. A majority of therapists heat the glass with a fire source and then place the glass on the area affected. The heat creates an energy that draws out the toxic substances while lifting the skin. Some therapists utilize the use of a vacuum or pump in order to raise the skin and muscles.

The cupping therapy draws out stagnant, old, and inactive blood. It also brings it to the skin's surface that can create visible marks. If there's no stagnation within the affected area The marks are usually quite light and will disappear rapidly, but in the event of injuries, muscles that are rigid or illness, or you live a life of sedentary it is likely that you will see dark cupping marks following the treatment. The patterns and colors of the marks can vary based on the extent of stagnation of the affected area.

The marks of cupping look slightly scary, but the procedure is secure when done by qualified experts.

Chapter 2: The Benefits Of Cupping

There are many who remain skeptical about the advantages of cupping. Apart from a study conducted of cupping in China during the 50s, there have been numerous studies being conducted to test the effectiveness of cupping when it comes to alleviating muscle pain and improving the performance of athletes.

A study conducted by Hossam Metwally has shown dry and wet cupping techniques work well in the treatment of myofascial pain syndrome. The study involved 42 patients who were suffering of myofascial injury. They had not been previously treated with cupping therapy. The patients received cupping twice per week for 10 consecutive weeks. The results were astonishing. After 10 months, the team discovered that patients all noticed improvements and improved mobility. However, those suffering from neck pain or upper back pain saw the most improvement. Many patients continued using cupping after 10 weeks of cupping therapy because it made patients feel better.

There have been 725 clinical studies that were conducted regarding the efficacy of cupping treatment from 1958 until 2011, which includes 419 case series as well as 30 clinically controlled trials, and 163 random controlled studies. Studies have shown that cupping therapy may alleviate signs of herpes zoster and muscle pain, and many other ailments.

Cupping therapy has numerous proven advantages, such as:

It helps eliminate toxins in the body.

A diet that is a mixture of processed foods, eating in excess or not exercising enough, stress, dehydration, a poor diet and constipation could result in toxic build-up. If you're suffering from too many contaminants, you'll frequently feel exhausted. Also, you're prone to obesity and weight gain. The buildup of toxic substances can cause skin rashes, acne, muscle problems, bad breath weight gain as well as lower back pain. breast pain, fatigue and intolerance to fat-rich foods and flatulence, diarrhea and lower the resistance against infections.

Sports cupping improves blood circulation throughout your body, and increases the flow of blood that is fresh.

* This assists in flushing out all toxins within the body, and can treat ailments which are caused by accumulation of toxic waste, including aches as well as allergies, fevers poor circulation, anxiety, muscles pain, coughs, colds and the flu.

Cupping therapy can help athletes recover from intense training. Overtraining can lead to stress, which may lead to the accumulation of toxic waste in muscles.

It helps with anxiety and depression.

Depression and anxiety can impact people of all ages and include sports stars. Depression can lead to fatigue during the day and may affect one's physical performance.

Cupping therapy can help reduce symptoms of anxiety and depression through relaxing and detoxifying the body. It eliminates impurities, dead cells, toxins, and other toxins out of the human body. It carries oxygen-rich and fresh blood. The majority of therapists employ a mix of fixed and wet cupping. It typically takes six sessions to relieve anxiety and depression. Cupping can help restore wellbeing as well as happiness and emotional well-being by restoring equilibrium in the body.

It helps with many health issues.

If you're a professional athlete you must ensure your body is healthy every day. Simple health issues like fever, flu or a bacterial infection could affect your performance.

Cupping can alleviate and treat various health issues common to everyone like common colds, asthma allergies, infections asthma IBS gastritis and diarrhea abdominal pain, fatigue acne, hiccups blood pressure, arthritis migraine, stomach pain and migraine.

Cupping therapy is also able to treat many more serious illnesses such as diabetes mellitus asthma bronchial, acne, heart diseases Carpal tunnel syndrome, facial palsy, chest pain hemorrhoids, hernias, anxiety, paralysis, cough depression, back pain and fibromyalgia. and gout. But, certain claims aren't supported by studies conducted by scientists. For serious ailments, always consult a doctor or specialist in the area.

In addition, it helps treat ailments that impact athletic performance, like over-training syndrome, inflammation, muscles cramps that are caused by exercise as well as asthma, plantar fasciitis heat stroke, Rhabdomyolysis.

It boosts performance in sports.

Our bodies aren't without limits. For those who are athletes you're stretching your body beyond the limit. It is able to provide quick relief from muscle strain and reduces the effects of the muscle strain. It can improve sports performance in a variety of ways. It relaxes muscles that are tight and adhesions. It actually pulls adhesions away and relaxes muscles that are tight.

It also enhances your sporting performance through the increase in blood flow. Insufficient blood circulation can affect your endurance and energy. It can cause muscle pain and cramps that may limit your performance and mobility. There is also hair loss and varicose veins. It can also cause lower leg pain, infections shortness of breath, headache, dizziness, edema foot ulcers, as well as variations in temperature of the skin. Cupping can improve circulation of blood by drawing the skin in the cup. It draws blood to the region, allowing the fluid to circulate more readily and accelerate the repair of damaged tissue.

Cupping is a treatment for the most frequent problems that athletes face, including muscles spasms, plantar fasciitis and chronic muscle imbalances. shoulder pain, joint back pain and neck pain.

Cupping in sports naturally improves endurance and agility. It boosts endurance, speed as well as concentration, mobility, and stamina.

It encourages relaxation.

Training for sports can be stressful, physically as well as mentally. Stress can be more harmful than you imagine. It can affect your immune system and come with a variety of signs like headaches, depressed energy, a loss of passion for sexual activity, chest pains as well as a rapid heart rate as well as social isolation, frequent illnesses, pessimism, as well as the inability to concentrate. Cupping therapy eases anxiety by eliminating the toxins that are in the body and allowing energy or qi flow freely. Cupping helps balance the distribution of blood and energy in your body, enhancing the efficiency of your organs as well as alleviating stress.

The cupping therapy is economical and secure. It improves more than flexibility and improves the elasticity of muscles. It also improves your overall health and standard of life too. It helps you relax and provides you with the energy to complete the activities you've always wanted to accomplish.

Chapter 3: The Different Types Of Cupping Therapy

Cupping has been practiced for centuries It's not surprising that there are a variety of cupping therapies. Each cupping method is created to accomplish a particular objective. For instance dry cupping is primarily used to release the adhesions between muscles and the fascia. The wet cupping method however can be used to eliminate the toxins.

Dry cupping is the most popular method utilized to treat a variety of ailments in the West while wet cupping is the method that is used in the middle east.

Here's a list of different types of cupping therapy: (this section is fine however it requires refinement. Eliminate the moderate, weak and the weak cupping techniques and classify them according to intensity. In dry cupping, put the vacuum flash, empty or massage. Under water, place herbs or water.

Different types of cups

Dry Cupping

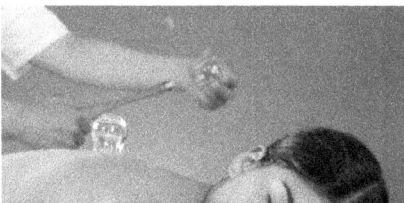

Dry cupping may be the most fundamental cupping method. It's also known as fire cupping. The therapist warms the cup by using fire, and then swiftly place the cup onto the skin of the patient. The heat draws blood and lifts the skin upwards. The air in cups creates vacuum, which increases the redness and expansion of the skin. The cup sits upon the face for 5-10 minutes. Most therapists prefer the glass cup for dry cupping since they're stronger and simple to sterilize.

This method of cupping is secure and will not cause any discomfort. It's just a brief squeeze sensation.

Wet Cupping

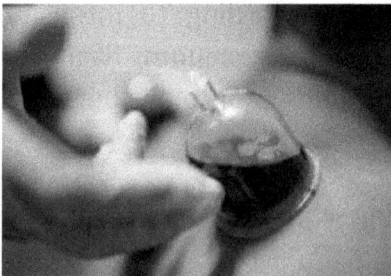

Wet cupping is one of the most commonly used cupping technique. This type of cupping is called Hijama and is popularly employed throughout Middle Eastern countries. Middle East. The therapist places a hot cup over the skin of the patient and allows it to sit for between 5 and 10 minutes while allowing the cup raise the skin. After that, he takes off the cup, and then employs a knife or scalpel to create small cuts on the area affected. Then, he places another cup over the cut and then uses a pump to draw the blood that is toxic out and raise the skin. The therapist removes the cup, and then applies the bandage and antibiotic ointments on the skin to stop infections.

This technique is definitely bloody, however it's a little uncomfortable. Patients will feel an immediate pinching sensation as a result of the cut. However, there's no reason to be concerned. The incisions heal in short amount of time and do not leave marks. If you are suffering from an inability to tolerate pain and are unable to tolerate pain, you may ask your specialist to use local anesthesia.

Massage Cupping

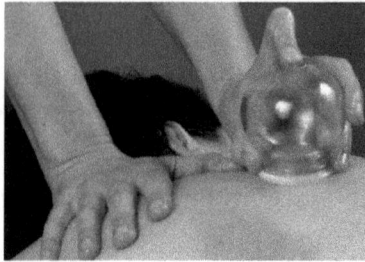

This is a kind of dry cupping. It is sometimes referred to as massage cupping. The therapist rubs essential oils to the skin, and then puts the cup on the affected region or the cupping point. When the suction has begun the therapist will move the cup across the skin. This results in an inverse massage effect. Instead of applying pressure on various massage points on the body to help heal this method uses suction to pull the tissues, muscles, and the skin upwards. This is a powerful treatment for weight loss and healing that chiropractors have used for years as well as physical therapy and spa treatments.

Massage cupping increases circulation of blood to tissues and muscles. It relaxes muscles and releases tightness and adhesions. It also relieves chronic congestion. The cupping therapy method is so soothing that the patient could be able to fall asleep.

Flash Cupping

If you're trying to minimize your appearance with marks it's recommended to go with this method. Flash cupping is a method used to apply short-interval suction or flashes. The therapist spreads herbs and healing creams to the body. He heats the cup with an open flame and then puts it onto the face for approximately five minutes. Then, he removes the cup and puts it back on the skin for another five minutes. This procedure is repeated numerous times. This technique is utilized for cupping the face as well as other areas of the body.

Herbal Cupping

This method of cupping is employed to treat neck shoulder pain, shoulder pain cough, asthma and the common cold. The method employs a variety of tools like clamps made of metal or fire, water, herbs, a deep pans bamboo cups. Bamboo cups and herbs are placed in boiling water bath for around 30 minutes before being applied on the skin. The therapist generally employs a variety of Chinese herbs , such as lotsus seed, astralagus

Ganoderma or lingzhi, dang Gui or angelica sinesis ma huang, ephedra sinica as well as licorice root and the gingko biloba plant, the lily bulbs, flowers of honeysuckle, isatis along with perilla leaf.

Water Cupping

This is a complex procedure which should be carried out by an experienced practitioner. The therapist puts 3/4 cup of water inside the glass, and then quickly puts the cup onto the skin, making sure not to spill the water. This method is utilized to treat dry coughs, asthma or rheumatism. It also relieves discomfort.

Needle Cupping

This is also referred to as cupping of acupuncture. The needle is placed on the acupuncture points. After that the cup is positioned at the location in which the needle is. This method is employed to boost the effects of acupuncture. It is beneficial to athletes. This method relieves neck pain and sciatica, stroke, joint pains, biliary, chronic fatigue, hypertension fasciitis and fibromyalgia. the morning sickness syndrome, kidney colic Rheumatoid arthritis as well as allergic rhinitis. The technique can also treat various illnesses like insomnia, hyperlipaemiaand neurodermatitis, lactation, obesity, Raynaud syndrome, reflex sympathetic dystrophy, vascular dementia ulcerative colitis, urolithiasis sore throat, tourette syndrome as well as hepatitis, herpes osteoarthritis and female infertility.

Techniques for Cupping based on the Intensity

• Weak cupping

Based on the name, this method offers soft pressure. The suction is accomplished by altering the dimensions of the flame or by pulling the pump gun gently. The result is usually a slight pink circle which will fade within a few hours.

This method of cupping is used to aid in relaxing the body and increase circulation. It assists in healing by improving circulation of the body. It is classified as a gentle cupping treatment that is offered to those who are younger than 7 years old or older. The treatment could be for as long as 30 minutes. It is recommended for mild health problems like asthma, colds tonsillitis, sore throat, and sore throat.

* Medium Cupping:

This method uses suction or medium pressure. The suction is strong and might feel uncomfortable initially. The suction will cause visible bruises or marks.

It is the most commonly used treatment for people with strong Chi. It is to be safe for children older than 7 years old to undergo this specific treatment. The treatment duration is 15 minutes. It can be utilized to treat migraines, injuries from sports, and the stress-related disorders.

"Strong Cupping."

The cupping method is distinguished by a powerful suction that can drain the Chi. It is typically used to cleanse and can leave dark bruises following the treatment. According to Chinese medical practices, these bruises are caused by toxins eliminated from blood and the body. This is the kind of cupping used for chronic musculoskeletal issues.

Myofascial Decompression Therapy

Myofascial compression therapy is more popularly referred to as cupping for sports. It is a traditional Chinese cupping therapy targets twelve meridians that run through the body to help heal. Myofascial decompression therapy in contrast is targeted at the muscular and skeletal system of the body. While, many sports cupping therapists use Acupuncture points. The method typically uses mechanical vacuum machine to create suction. The cup is connected to a suction machine and placed on the skin. The therapist will usually massage the patient using cream and herbal oils prior to placing the cup onto the skin.

This technique of cupping is employed to:

* Reduce myofascial pain and poor patterning because of hypertonic muscles

Reduce scar adhesions, scar tissue, as well as myofascial dysfunction.

* Reduce the amount of tender and hypersensitive tissues, also known as trigger points.

Myofascial decompression therapy is not painful, however it may cause bruises, which would fade within a few days. The pressure applied by suction improves the flexibility of tissues and reduces swelling. It is used to treat many injuries to athletes, including tendon injuries, workout injuries and tail bone injuries. muscle soreness, shinsplints and rotator cuff tears, the groin, head injuries and concussions. Sciatica is an Achilles tendon injuries, as well as dislocated shoulders. We'll go over more in depth later.

Chapter 4: Who Provides Cupping Therapy?

It is usually safe when performed by a certified professional. The method of healing is typically used by chiropractors, doctors or acupuncturists as well as physical therapists. A large number of massage therapists and sports coaches are also certified to provide this kind of therapy.

There are many certification programs and courses that deal with sports cupping and cupping in general that include:

ACE Massage Cupping

This course provides the certificate necessary to use massage cupping. The 2017 edition of this course costs around $140.

The Best Cure and Care

The institute is in the UK however, it also offers courses at level 4 for therapists across the world. The students will receive a diploma as well as an official certificate upon completion of the course. The cost of this certification course is PS650. After you have completed the course, you are able to join of both the General Regulatory Council for

Complementary Therapies (GRRCT) as well as BCS (British Cupping Society).

Hijama Cupping Certification Course

The certification course was designed by the Director of the Hijama Clinic and is available to both male and female students. It can be completed in just a few hours and cost about PS475.

Hijama Training Institute

The Institute offers an online, level 5 or higher Diploma Hijama class. This is a program that is completed in about 400 hours. This course covers an overview of the origins and history behind cupping as well as cupping methods and the anatomy of human anatomy. It also provides hands-on course. This course costs about PS475.

Modern Cupping Methods, Certification Program

The training takes place across various regions in North America, Europe, Canada as well as Asia. It provides both theoretical and practical training. Students are able to test their skills with seven different cups. Students who successfully have completed the training will earn the certification of Contemporary

Cupping Therapy. The course is three days long which costs about $690.

It is crucial to place your security first. If you choose to try this alternative therapy ensure that it is performed by a qualified and accredited professional.

Chapter 5: The Way To Do Sports Cupping

Cupping in sports is the secret weapon used by elite athletes. It appears to be difficult and intimidating however, it's actually simple to perform:

Cupping Tools

In order to begin you'll require some tools, such as:

Cups

You can make use of a standard cup, but if would like to get the most result from your treatment, you should make use of special myofascial decompression cups.

Bamboo cup - The are used to make herbal cupping. These cups are not expensive however, you must polish them with sandpaper before use to eliminate rough edges. The edges of the cup need to be smooth. Bamboo is a disadvantage. cups is that they're prone to cracking. This can lead to air leaks which weaken the suction.

Suction cups Suction cups are utilized for cupping in sports and are typically constructed of plastic. They are durable, easy to break and safe. These cups are usually connected with a suction device or pump. suction device.

Glass cups The cups are shaped as the shape of a ball. They are available in a variety of sizes, including small, medium and large. They are sturdy as well as easy to wash.

Facial cups - These facial cups are typically small and have round pumps.

There are many cup sizes available such as:

Diameter of the Cup or Code

1 Six centimeters by one

Two centimeters by one

Three centimeters by Four Centimeters

Four One-by-3 centimeters

Five One By Two and Half Centimeters

Six centimeters by one inch

At a minimum, you'll need six cups #1. Then, purchase perhaps four cups of the cup number 2 or #3.

Vacuum Suction Pump There are a variety of suction vacuum pumps. The most inexpensive one is the plastic handheld pump, which costs around $0.50. There are also several an electric power press available. It typically costs $38.47.

Essential Oils

Aromatherapy can enhance the effects of cupping for sports. To reap the maximum benefits of cupping, you should diffuse essential oils like:

Lavenderis a remedy for muscle spasms, cramps arthritis, and sprains. It also helps ease anxiety and stress.

Marjoram is a vital oil that treats spasms, and relieves anxiety and stress. It is often referred to as the "happy herb.

Wintergreen Oil - This one has an anti-inflammatory and anti-spasmodic impact. It's a natural cure to treat muscle spasms and cramps. spasms, headaches and muscles pains.

Eucalyptus The essential oil is a wonder for athletes. It's extremely relaxing and can ease nerve pain as well as fibrosis.

Peppermint Oil - This oil helps relieve muscle cramps, pains, and soreness. It is a potent anti-inflammatory with anti-spasmodic qualities.

Clary Sage - This vital oil helps ease headaches, breathing cramps muscles spasms, and headaches.

Roman chamomile - It is an effective antispasmodic oil with strong healing capabilities.

Ginger Essential oil - This oil helps reduce stiffness and pain. It eases joint pains tension, tendonitis, and spasms.

Rosemary It is an oil for relaxation that helps improve memory. It cleanses the liver, and assists in relieving anxiety.

Ointments: You'll require antibiotic creams to cleanse your skin as well as treat any blisters. This is particularly true during cupping with water.

Needles

If you're considering combining acupuncture and cupping, you'll require a set of top quality needles for acupuncture.

You can locate some of these instruments in stores selling medical supplies however, you can also locate a variety of high-quality cupping sets on marketplaces online like eBay or Amazon.

BASIC CUPPING

Step 1

Clean the cups before using them with salt water. Make sure that the cups are dry and clean prior to making use of them. It is not recommended to reuse the same cup. It is recommended to use a different set of cups for each patient, or ask them to get their own for exclusive use. If you're using glass cups they can be sterilized so that they can be reused.

Step 2

Examine the patient's complaints and signs of disease by looking at the signs. After identifying the illness then you have to determine the cupping points associated with that specific medical disease. For instance, if you suffer from neck pain, then it is necessary to put the cups on your back and both sides of your spine.

Step 3.

The client should lie down face-down. To prevent infection, clean your cupping areas. Cleanse the skin using the soapy water. After that, apply natural oil or cream to the skin.

Step 4

Connect an air pump onto the cup. Then, put it on your skin. Press the pump until it creates suction. Take the pump off, and then put a Cup on top of the skin.

You can employ the method of fire cupping in case you don't have a cupping pump. Put a cotton ball into the cup of pure alcohol. Then, you can remove the ball of cotton from its cup with the forceps of a pair, and ignite the cotton ball with matches. The lids of the glass cups with the fire. After that, you can quickly put the cups on the skin. Make sure to check the suction, and be sure it's not painful or uncomfortable.

Step 5

After all the cups are set There are many ways to approach the treatment. This will differ based according to the health of the patient. At first, you may apply static cupping to the painful areas and cupping points. To help your muscles recover after a workout it is also possible to perform the massage or moving cupping.

Step 6

In the next 10 mins, request that the patient lie down. After that, take the cups off. Clean the marks or blisters by using alcohol or antibiotic application.

It can take several days before the signs disappear. Treatment with cups to treat an injury or muscle condition is recommended twice per week for a couple of weeks. Check the condition regularly of the muscles prior to providing the treatment. When the muscles are fully recovered treatments can be stopped or reduced depending on the need.

Massage Cupping

Massage cupping basically adds motion to your cupping routine. The primary reason behind this type of therapy is to stimulate the lymphatic system and to increase blood flow. Although this is regarded as an intense massage, it does not require similar effort to regular massage. If used to aid in the post-workout or recovery from exercise The treatment works by relaxing the fascia as well as dislodging any accumulation of fluids within the tissues.

This method typically uses one cup at a given time. It is modified according to your body part you wish to work.

You'll need:

* Cupping set

The essential oil can be used in conjunction with any other lotion of your choice

1. Request that the client lay down on the flat surface. It could be a massage bed or any other comfortable mattress that promotes

relaxation and is suitable to perform the procedure.

2. Apply oil lightly on the area you wish to treat. It is recommended to apply therapeutic oils which aid in the therapeutic effect. The oil aids in helping to make it easier to move the cups.

3. Make sure the clean cups are placed near the bed. Most often, just 1 cup can be used at any one time , but it can be different in size depending on the location of treatment.

4. Set the cup at the exact cupping point. When you're working with a cupping setup that includes the pump gun as well as a pipe, connect the pipe to both the pump gun and the cup. This set of cupping is more suitable to massage cupping because it's more consistent. If the cup shatters during massage, you can pump it up to return the vacuum. But, you are able to make use of any cupping device you own.

5. Create a vacuum by using an air pump in order to hold the cup. If you have a cupping set with vacuum nozzles, simply turn it clockwise to create a vacuum, then twist it counterclockwise to let it release.

6. Make sure you are not uncomfortable and uncomfortable. The cups should be moved slowly in an outward direction or away from the center of your body or towards your lower extremities. If you find places where the cups aren't able to move, don't push it. For practitioners who are certified such stops are usually an indication that there's blockage in your area, and additional work must be carried out to alleviate those. The skin of the cup is evaluated prior to beginning. Continue to massage for 5 and 10 minutes during the initial session.

7. The suction can be released by pressing just under the rim of cup when using the pump gun for cupping sets. Massage cupping is usually not a cause of any marks since it rarely is left in place for very long. But, it can depend on the health of the patient as well as the professional who administers the treatment.

Be aware that the steps above are taken from my book the Basics of Cupping.

Myofascial Decompression Therapy

Take note that this procedure is best performed by an authorized professional. The reason for this is because they have a thorough and proven understanding of the theories that guide the practice that is a blend of muscle physiology as well as the meridians in the body. The process described in this article are general, and differs depending on the location in which there has been an injury or muscle strain.

What should you expect during your treatment?

The physician will determine the signs and the location of the issue. Exercises in range of motion (ROM) will be conducted to identify the muscles involved and for guidance following treatment. These ROM exercises will continue throughout the treatment. Patients will be required to stretch and flex various muscle groups while the cups are placed

What to expect following the procedure:

Muscles are strained and weak caused by active stretching and flexion of various muscles.

Items required:

Sets of cups (preferable vacuum cups to make it easy for attachment and release)

Cream or oil

Procedure:

1. The client should be placed in a position that is based on the muscle group that is targeted.

2. Massage the area with oil for better adhesion of the cups. Optional: The doctor can offer massage cupping at first to help calm the patient and relax the muscles.

3. Apply the cups along Meridian lines that cross the muscle groups that are targeted or on the muscle group that is affected or adhesions scarred.

4. Perform the range of motion exercises when the cups are securely attached. It varies based on the muscles and the specific game that the client participates in. For those who run, the therapist may ask the client to imitate the movements of muscles when they're running, such as hip flexions and extension. For swimmers, this could be a pull and reach move as if swimming.

5. Take the cups off.

6. Examine the areas, and then examine the data from before and the results of post-treatment.

Chapter 6: The Cupping Points

Which body part should you be able to cup? The answer is based on your medical conditions and the type of cupping therapy you are employing. There are various cupping points within the body, as shown in the image below. Each point is able to treat specific ailments.

F2 - toothache, deafness and sore eyes.

F4 - sinusitis, facial paralysis, trigeminal neuralgia, blocked nose

The mouth is a source of ulceration facial paralysis, toothache jaw pain

Dry mouth tonsillitis, mumps

The TH4 is asthma cough, bronchitis pneumonia

TH1 - pharyngitis, bronchitis, asthma, vocal cord problems, hoarse voice

Th6 - jaundice, hepatitis, an enlarged gallstones, liver

TH7 - cardiac spasms, heart problems

TH8 - heart valve issues or cardiac spasm

TH2 - insufficient lactation, bronchial spasm, chest pain

A3 - Hepatitis, an enlarged liver

The TH5 causes chest pain, Ischemia, cardiac spasm

TH2 - chest pain, mastitis, bronchial asthma, insufficient lactation

The TH3C virus causes chest pain as well as asthmatic bronchial

F3- rhinitis, vertigo, sinusitis, dizziness

Hi face paralysis, migraine eye strain, trigeminal neurogia, eye pressure

LE15- arthritis

LE14 - the groins are itchy, endometriosis

L6: knee pain problems with the knee cap the knee joint, thigh discomfort

L13 - liver issues irregular menstrual flow, urinary incontinence

A7- irregular menstruation, ovarian dysfunction, appendicitis, infertility

LE11 Le11 - abnormal uterine bleeding irregular menstrual cycle, wet dreams and dysmenorrhea

LE12 - irregular menstrual flow bleeding from the uterus, menstrual cramps

LE13 - liver issues and kidney issues and urinary incontinence. menstrual flow

A8 - endometriosis, irregular menstruation, cystitis, hernia

LE8 - uterine bleeding and menstrual irregularities

The LE7 kneecap issues Thigh pain, hip pain and knee pain

A4- diabetes and an enlarged spleen

A5- kidney stones, constipation, kidney dysfunction, kidney pain

UE3 Shoulder pain

A1 - peptic ulcers, gastritis, bloated stomach, vomiting, indigestion, hiccups

A6- irregular menstrual cycle appendicitis and vaginal discharge

The cupping points that are used are known as Tibb Cupping Points which are only suitable if you're employing the dry cupping method.

Hijama Cupping Point

Hijama is a cupping method that draws blood by small incisions on the skin. This technique was developed by Hippocrates and was practiced across various countries in the time of ancient times, such as Greece, Saudi Arabia, Persia as well as Turkey. There are various cupping points used in hijama, as seen in the images below:

Figure 1.1 Cupping points on the back, which includes the head

Figure 1.2 Cupping points located in at the top of the body which includes those on the sides of your face.

Figure 1.3 Cupping points at the side of your body, including the face

Chapter 7: The Trigger Points And Cupping

As we mentioned previously Cupping can help release scar tissue adhesions forming between the fascia and the muscle and improves mobility. Also, it releases trigger points.

Trigger points are painful muscle band that connects the myofascia muscle to the muscle. Trigger points typically occur in the back, neck and shoulder muscles when the muscles are stressed for prolonged durations of time. Trigger points can create discomfort and serious problems for athletes. They can impede movement by keeping muscles short and stiff. These points trigger muscles contractions that may cause nerve entrapment.

In addition to in addition to the Tibbs as well as the Hijama Cupping Points cups can also be applied directly to trigger points to alleviate the pain of muscles and improve mobility. The suction of the cup causes an unfavourable pressure on the area affected and stretch the thickened fascia muscles, and enhancing the athlete's movements.

There are many trigger points throughout the body, such as:

1. Subclavius - It is a tiny triangular muscle that lies within the first rib, and clavicle.

2. Pectoralis major is an oblong muscle that is located in the chest area. It is the largest of the chest muscles.

3. Pectoralis minor - It is a small muscle that lies in the upper portion of your chest. It is just below the pectoralis main.

4. Sternalis The sternalis is situated directly in front of pectoralis major and runs directly parallel to the border of the sternum.

5. Anterior Deltoid - This muscle is responsible for the rounded shape that your shoulders have. The anterior deltoid can also be called front delts.

6. Serratus anterior This is a saw form muscle found within your rib region.

7. Triceps: The triceps is a muscle with a lot of mass situated on the lower back of the upper leg. The triceps is the muscle responsible for extension the elbow joint. It lets you straighten your arms.

8. Biceps - It is a muscle found in the upper arm, between your shoulder and elbow. It is utilized when lifting things, and it is often used in exercises for strength.

9. Palmaris longus - It is a spindle-like muscle situated near your palms. you typically use it to turn your wrist.

10. Pronator Teres - The pronator Teres is situated in the forearm. It is used to rotate your forearms in order to feel your palms.

11. External Oblique - The external Oblique is located within your abdomen and is the largest muscle in the anterior lateral abdomen. It is connected to the subcostal and thoracoabdominal nerves. It is the one responsible for the torso's rotation. body.

12. McBurney's Point - This muscle is located on the right-hand side of your abdomen. If this region is tender, it's an indication that you have acute appendicitis.

13. Adductor longus The muscle is located in the thigh. It is able to flex your hip joint . It's responsible for the adduction and flexion of your hips.

14. The Gracilis is a superficial muscle situated on the medial side of the thigh. The muscle

rotates medially as it adducts, rotates, and flexes the hip.

15. Levator scapulae: The muscle rotates and raises your scapula. It's located to the rear and on the side of your neck.

16. The upper trapezius is one of two major muscles of the superficial which is located from the occipital bone all the way to below thoracic vertebrae. The muscle rotates, retracts the scapula, depresses, and lifts the scapula.

17. Supraspinatus - This muscles is located in the back of your upper part. It is located at the shoulder's back and just below your neck.

18. Iliocostalis Thoracis is located in the rib area and is utilized to stretch and flex your vertebral column, both unilaterally and bilaterally.

19. Infraspinatus The infraspinatus is a strong triangular muscle that can rotate and stabilize the arm. It's located in the rear of your shoulder.

20. Teres Minor - This is a small and elongated muscle found in the rotator the cuff. Laterally, it rotates arms and stabilizes the humerus.

21. Rhomboids The rhomboids connect the upper end of vertebral column. It rotates medially and pulls the scapulae.

22. Lower trapezius - This area is frequently referred to"the "bitchy spot" by chiropractors who are registered. It's on the left-hand side that runs along your back. It rotates and adducts the scapula. Lower trapezius fibers contain trigger points or TrPs which cause pain in the upper cervical region. The trigger points could cause headaches as well.

23. Gluteus Maximus - The muscles rotates in a lateral direction and may extend hip joints. The muscle also extends your hip while abducting the hips. It is utilized for various exercises, like dead lifts, kettlebell swings and squats the hip thrust, reverse hyperextension and glute-ham raises.

24. Iliopsoas is the result of the union of two muscles: the iliacus and the psoas major. The abdominal region is where it's located, and it runs through the thighs. It flexes the hips , and is believed as the most powerful of the hip flexors.

25. Erector spinae - The spinae is comprised of three long and thin muscles that run along either side of the vertebral column. The

muscles are known as spinalis, longissimus and iliocostalis.

26. The gracilis the strap-line muscles which runs between the pubic bone and on the other side of knees. It is able to rotate and flex your leg in the medial direction. The thigh also gets adducted.

27. Adductor Longus - This is a muscle in the skeletal system that is situated in the lower thigh. It is adducts the thigh as well as the hip. It also allows the hip joint to flex. If the muscle is stressed it will cause tension, pain or discomfort in the region.

28. Sartorius muscles - Sartorius - Sartorius muscles is small muscle that runs across the thighs. It is located between the anterior and upper portion of the thigh. Its name comes by the Latin word meaning tailor. It's also referred to as the tailor's muscle.

29. Piriformis is a pear-shaped muscle which is found in the gluteal area of your leg. It's located in the pelvis, right above the buttocks.

30. Hamstrings Hamstrings are muscles that are located behind your thigh. They flex the knees as well as extends your hips.

31. Biceps femoris : The biceps fascia is beneath the Hamstrings. Laterally, it rotates as it extends, flexes, and rotates the knee joints.

32. The Quadratus Lumborum Deep is located in the spine region. It is a trigger spot that plays an important part in the progression of hip pain related problems as well as lower back pain that is chronic and sciatica-related symptoms.

33. Gastrocnemius is located in the back of the leg's lower part. It is a significant muscle of the calf. It is a double-joint muscle that flexes the knees as well as the foot. The overuse of this muscle could result in Achilles tendon pain.

34. Soleus - This muscles is found in the lower calf. This muscle is used when you're standing or walking. If the fascia that surrounds the soleus gets thicker it will cause the compartment syndrome , an illness that causes blood clots, neuropathy and atrophy of muscles.

35. Extensor longus digitorum - This is a pennate muscle situated in front of the leg

just above your feet. This muscle extends the toes.

36. Vastus medialis is an extensor muscle situated in your thigh. It is responsible for extending your knees. If this muscle is overstressed and over worked, it will suffer knee pain.

37. Tibialis anterior Tibialis anterior - This muscle is situated close to the shin, and is accountable for the inversion as well as doing the dorsiflexion in the feet. In the event of overuse, this muscle may limit your movements over time.

If you feel pain at the trigger points, then you could place the cup on them directly. Cupping them on trigger points will increase circulation of blood in the area, increasing its flexibility. muscles. This increases mobility and can also enhance sports performance.

Chapter 8: Acupuncture And Cupping

Therapy

Acupuncture is a well-known Traditional Chinese Medicine technique in which skilled therapists insert tiny needles through the skin. It is used to treat various ailments like muscle spasms, neck discomfort, osteoarthritis, allergies depression, knee pain. As with cupping therapy Acupuncture improves one's health through enhancing the flow Qi and blood in the body. Cupping and acupuncture are utilized in conjunction to treat various ailments.

Acupuncture points are the area of your body that you put the needle. The acupuncture points were designed to be a representation of how many days of the year. At first there were the 365 points of acupuncture. The points were then mapped to 14 acupuncture channel lines. There was a channel for each Organ, with one channel channel along the stomach's midline and one that runs along the spine. In time there were acupuncture spots that increased to about 2 000.

Each acupuncture point is linked with a list with diseases they treat. These acupuncture points can also be employed in sports cupping, which is why it's crucial to know these points.

There are 14 Acupuncture channels. These include the heart, large intestine, lung the pericardium, the small intestine, triple heater gall bladder, kidney stomach, liver, spleen, urinary tract and conception vessel, the governing vessel, as well as other points.

The distance between two points are measured by cun which is the length of the thumb's knuckle.

Lungs

The LU1 Zhongfu - This is situated on your left shoulder . it can stop cough and later stage lung disease. It's measured at 6 cuns away from the sternum.

LU2 Yunmen It is located one cun higher than the LU1. It helps stop cough.

The LU3 Tianfu It regulates ascending and declining of the vital energy qi. If this area has been blocked you'll feel the symptoms of drowsiness, coughing and breathlessness nosebleeds and goiter.

The LU4 Xiabai is located on the upper arm , and beneath the armpit. This regulates the flow of qi within the cun differences

LU5 Chize- This is located in the brachi tendon of the biceps. It helps to reduce the heat in the lungs and allows waterways to flow. It also helps to eliminate the phlegm that builds up in the lungs.

The LU6 Kongzui - You'll see this acupuncture spot on the wrist. It regulates lung qi.

The LU7 Lieque situated just above the wrist. It allows the nose to open and eliminates the phlegm. The distance is 0.5 cun space between LU7 and.

The LU8 Jingqu The LU8 Jingqu is just above the wristcrease, and is targeted at the throat and lungs.

The LU9 Taiyuan The area is situated on the right side of the radial artery close to the wrist. It's situated one cun lower than the LU8. It also has 7 cuns between the two.

It is LU10 Yuji - It relieves lung heat and reduces the cough. It also relaxes the mind.

LU11 Shaoshang - It's situated in the thumbnail's first the radial corner. It can open the orifices, and it targets the throat.

Large Intestine

LI1 Shangyang The Shangyang is located on the radial end the index finger. It is targeted at the throat and shoulder. It improves the brightness of your eyes and helps to snuff out the inner wind.

LI2 Erjian It is located above LI1.

LI3 Sanjian - It is situated on the top of LI2.

LI4 Hegu It is situated between the index finger and thumb. It is situated on the the top of LI3.

LI5 Yangxi It is situated at the wrist.

LI6 Pianli - This acupuncture spot is located at the LI5's top with a 3 cuns of distance between.

LI7 Wenliu is responsible for the regulation of the digestive tract. It's situated about 5 cuns above the wrist.

LI8 Xialian is located four cuns below the fold of your elbow.

LI9 Shanglian- You can locate this acupuncture point just above the LI8, just below the elbow, and one cun over the LI8.

LI10 Shousanli – This is located just under the elbow. just 1 cun of LI9.

LI11 Quchi - It is located near the elbow joint, 2 cuns above LI10.

LI12 Zhouliao The acupuncture point is located above the elbow , and it is targeted at the arms. It is situated 1 cun away from LI11.

LI13 Shouwuli – This can be found three cuns below the elbow's crevice. It helps eliminate the phlegm. it loosens the tendon. It is located just 2 cuns away from LI12.

LI14 Binao The acupuncture LI14 Binao is situated at the lower portion of the deltoids. It eases tension in the tendons, and helps to eliminate stagnation of the Qi. It is targeted at the eyes, arms and shoulders.

LI15 Jianyu The location is just above the shoulder blade. It targets the arms as well as the shoulders.

LI 16 Jugu This is situated between the acromion and the scapular spine. It is able to disperse lumps, and aids in the treatment of duct obstruction syndrome.

LI17 Tianding is located to the right of your throat.

LI18 Futu The location is above L17.

LI19 Heliao It is located between the mouth and nose.

LI20 Yingxiang is situated next to the nose wings.

Stomach

ST1 Chengqi The ST1 Chengqi enlightens the eyes and eliminates the eye of heat. It concentrates on the face, mouth and eye. It is located beneath the eye.

ST2 Sibai ST2 Sibai just below ST1.

ST3 Juliao - This location is located beneath ST2.

ST4 Dicang It is located on the cheek below ST3.

ST5 Daying is situated below St4 and at the mouth.

ST6 Jiache. This acupuncture spot is located on the left end of your mouth.

ST7 Xiaguan This is located to the left to the front of your face adjacent to the ear.

ST8 Touwei is found in the head, over the ear.

The ST9 Renying is within the neck, beneath the chin.

ST10 Suitu - It is situated between ST11 and ST8. The qi in the throat is controlled and eliminates the wind from the throat.

ST11 Qishe It is located beneath the neck, close to the shoulders blade. It eliminates heat from the lung and the phlegm.

ST12 Quepen - This area is located at the top margin as well as at the center of the clavicle.

ST13 Qihu located below ST12.

ST14 Kufang located below ST13.

ST15 Wuyi ST15 Wuyi situated below ST14 and is within the line connecting the nipple's center with the clavicle.

ST16 Yingchuang It can be found in your chest region. This regulates the circulation Qi within the chest.

ST17 Ruzhong ST17 Ruzhong located in the breast area.

ST18 Rugen This area reduces the amount of edema and reduces cough.

ST19 Burong. This point is located in the rib region just below the chest.

ST20 Chengman The location is just below ST19.

ST21 Liangmen ST21 Liangmen situated beneath ST20.

ST22 Guanmen It is located just below ST21.

ST23 Taiyi. This acupuncture point is located beneath ST22. This point controls the digestive tract as well as stomach. It eliminates phlegm and helps relax the mind.

ST24 Huaroumen is one cun higher than the umbilicus. It regulates stomach and the intestines.

ST25 Tianshu The Tianshu is located 2 cuns to the lateral side of your belly button. The spleen is controlled by it stomach and the the intestine.

ST26 Wailing is located just one cun below the navel. It eliminates moisture and regulates the stomach.

ST27 Daju The Daju is situated under the navel, and it regulates the flow of qi.

ST28 Suidao ST28 Suidao - It is situated below the navel, and just below ST27.

ST29 Guilai is situated 1 cun lower than ST28.

ST30 Qichong - It's situated above the thigh and beneath ST29.

ST31 Biguan clears the obstruction in the duct and releases winds. This is located inside the leg.

ST32 Futu It is situated approximately six cuns higher than the knee.

ST33 Yinshi is just below ST32 and three cuns above the knee.

ST34 Liangqiu. This acupuncture point is located two points above the knee.

ST35 Dubi - This is within the knee and the cavity that is in the lateral direction towards the ligament.

ST36 Zusanli, which is beneath the knee and helps to improve the function of the stomach and spleen.

ST37 Shangjuxu. This regulates the stomach as well as the intestines. It is situated below the knee and over three cuns below the knee.

ST38 Tiaokou It is located below ST37.

ST39 Xiajuxu is located below ST38.

ST40 Fenglong It is located next to the ST38.

ST41 Jiexi - This is in the middle of the crease on the ankle.

ST42 Chongyang The ST42 Chongyang is situated below the ST42.

ST43 Xiangu It is situated at the top of the feet.

ST44 Neiting - This is just below ST44.

ST45 Lidui ST45 Lidui - This is in the 2nd foot.

Spleen

SP1 Yinbai It is located on the medial part of the big toe. This area reduces bleeding and regulates your spleen.

SP2 Dadu is situated over SP2 and controls the spleen. It helps clear the mind as well.

SP3 Taibai - This is just above SP2 and is near the heel. It is a strong spleen that regulates the intestinal tract.

SP4 Gongsun The SP4 Gongsun is located to the right on the bottom.

SP5 Shangui - It is situated at the bottom of the metatarsal bone just above the feet. It stops bleeding, and regulates menstrual flow and the intestines.

SP6 Sanyinjiao SP6 Sanyinjiao - This is situated on the posterior edge of the bone that is called the shin. This regulates both the liver as well as the spleen.

SP7 Logu It is located 6 cuns higher than the posterior border of the bone that runs from the hind shin. It targets the leg as well as the abdomen.

SP8 Diji - It is located 3 cuns below SP9. It cleanses and harmonizes the spleen. It also regulates the uterus.

SP9 Yinlingquan The location is on the left side that of knee. This regulates the spleen, and enhances the functioning of the urinary tract.

SP10 Xuehai is two cuns below that border on the left side of patella. It regulates menstrual cycle.

SP11 Jimen - This is in the back of the thigh.

SP12 Chongmen - This is near the pelvis region.

SP13 Fushe SP13 Fushe this acupuncture spot above SP12 on the left side of the pelvis region.

SP14 FujieThis is located beneath that navel region.

SP15 Daheng is located over SP14.

SP16 Fuai SP16 Fuai is located over SP 15.

SP17 Shidou - This is approximately 6 cun from the middle of the chest.

SP18 Tianxi It is directly above SP17.

SP19 Xiongxiang – This acupuncture point is situated just above SP19.

SP20 Zhourung - This is just below the shoulder blade, over SP 19

SP21 Dabao The SP21 Dabao is located on the side of the breast.

Heart

Jiquan HE1 - This is located within the armpit.

He2 Qingling It is located 3 cuns higher than the elbow.

HE3 Shaohai The location is within the elbow region. It relaxes the mind and helps clear channel obstructions.

Lingdao HE4 - This is over 1.5 cuns above the wrist.

He5 Tongli - This is just below the HE4.

HE6 Yinxi The point is lower than HE6.

Shenmen Shenmen is right next to the HE7.

The HE8 Shaofu - This is situated on the palm, at the the top of the pinky finger.

Shaochong HE9 - This can be found in the nail region that is located on the finger's pinky.

Small Intestine

SI1 Shaoze SI1 Shaoze near the nail region of the pinky finger.

SI2 Qiangu This is situated just above SI1.

SI3 Houxi. This point is located at the bottom of the pinky finger.

SI4 Wangu - It is situated on the ulnar aspect on the palm.

SI5 Yanggu The SI5 Yanggu point is situated in the ulnar part of transverse crease. It eliminates heat and also removes the humidity in the knees.

SI6 Yanglao. This is on the wrist.

SI7 Zhizheng - This is situated between the elbow and hand.

SI8 Xiaohai The SI8 Xiaohai is located in the elbow region. It is evident when you bend your elbow.

SI9 Jianzhen The SI9 Jianzhen is located at the top of the armpit.

SI10 Naoshu is located in the shoulder region.

SI11 Tianzhongshu. This point is located just below the shoulder blade.

SI12 Tianchuang It is located above of the shoulders blades. It is targeted at the scapula, shoulder and trapezius.

SI13 Quyuan - It is located at the far end of the supraspinal cavity in the scapula.

SI14 Jianwaishu SI14 Jianwaishu - This is situated in the levator muscle in the scapula.

SI15 Jianzhongshu is on the left side of the neck. Just below your ear.

SI16 Tianchung The SI16 Tianchung is located on the right side from the neck.

SI17 Rianrong It occurs in the jaw region. It releases heat and eliminates the dampness.

SI18 Quanliao – This is located inside the cheek.

SI19 TinggongIt is located close to the ear region.

Bladder

BL1 Jingming - This is situated between the nose and the eye.

The BL2 Zanzhu It is situated within the eyebrow region.

The BL3 Meichong is located in the middle of your scalp.

The BL4 Gucha The Gucha is situated next to BL4.

The BL5 Wuchu - This point is higher than BL5.

BL6 Chengguang This is located above your head, about 1.5 above the BL6.

The BL7 Tongtian The price is 1.5 cun higher than BL6.

Luoque BL8 is 1.5 cun more than BL7.

BL9 Yuzhen - This is situated on the rear of the head, close to the ear.

BL10 Tianzhu - This is located below BL9.

BL11 Dazhu The Dazhu is located just below the neck, right next to the shoulder blade.

The BL12 Fengmen - This point is also beneath the neck, just behind your shoulder blade.

Feishu BL13 is located above your chest.

Bl14 Jueyinshu This is located in the upper part on the chest.

BL15 Xinshu It is located in the middle of the chest.

BL16 Dushu - This regulates the heart . it is located in the middle of the chest.

BL17 Geshu - This is in the middle of the chest.

The BL18 Ganshu - This Acupuncture point is aligned with T9. It helps to reduce heat and brighten the eyes. It also helps to nourish blood.

The BL19 Danshu - This spot is leveled by T5 and lies in the middle of the rib region.

B20 Pishu - It is leveled using T11 and is situated just above the stomach area.

It is BL21 Weishu Acupuncture spot is located in the stomach region.

The BL22 Sanjiaoshu can be found in the stomach region. It is the one that opens up the waterway.

BL23 Shenshu - This acupuncture spot is situated in the stomach region just over the navel.

BL24 Qihaishu - This area lies in your stomach and strengthens that lower back. It also regulates menstrual flow.

The BL25 Dachangshu is situated about 1.5 cuns lateral to GV3 and at the same level as L4. It helps strengthen lower back muscles and increases functioning of the intestinal.

B26 Guanyuanshu This point helps strengthen lower back muscles and enhances the function of the urinary tract.

BL27 Xiaochangshu The location is in the pelvic region.

BL28 Pangguangshu - This is just below BL27.

29 Zhonglushu Acupuncture spot is below the BL28.

BL30 Baihuanshu It is located just below BL29.

BL31 Shangliao - This is situated in the middle of the pelvis and about 1.5 cun lateral from BL27.

Ciliao BL32 - This is just below the BL31.

The BL33 Zhongliao The acupuncture spot is located below the BL32.

The acupuncture spot is situated in the lower part of the pelvis and just below BL33.

B35 Huiyanglt is close to the bone of the tail.

The BL36 Chengfu It is just below the buttocks.

The BL37 Yinmen is about 6 cuns away from the BL36.

The BL38 Fuxi It is in the rear on the back of your knee.

It is BL39. Weiyang The acupuncture spot is below BL38.

BL40 Weizhong It is situated next to BL40.

BL41 Fufen The point is located three cuns from the midline of the spine.

The BL42 Pohu - This is situated near the spine border of the scapula.

Gaohuangshu BL43 - This feeds the spleen as well as the heart. It is located on the back of the upper part.

The BL44 Shentang It is situated just below BL44, and about 3 cuns from the GV11.

The BL45 Yixi is situated 3 cuns of the middle line. It eases cough and reduces the heat.

BL46 Geguan - This is situated in the back, and regulates the functions of stomach. It regulates the middle burner as well.

The BL47 Hunmen point is situated at the back of the body. It regulates Qi in the liver and enhances the performance that the tendon performs.

The BL48 Yanggang - This is 3 cuns from the midline. It reduces heat in the gallbladder.

The BL49 Yishe - This is located in the rear.

The BL50 Weicang This point is located 3 cun away off the centerline. It regulates qi and eases pain.

The BL51 Huangmen is only 3 cuns from the GV5.

BL52 Zhishi - This is 3 cun in laterality to the GV4. It can improve our urinary tract. It increases your endurance and back.

BL53 Baohuang - It is located in the buttocks region. It helps improve the function of the bladder.

The BL54 Zhibian - It's found in the sacral part of the body. It aids in the improvement of the urinary tract as well as helps treat hemorrhoids.

BL55 Heyang This is 2 cuns to the left of the popliteal line in the middle of your calves.

BL56 Chengjin The BL56 Chengjin is lower than the BL55. It is located in the calf region.

BL57 Chengshan It is located below the BL40. It relaxes the muscles and treats hemorrhoids.

The BL58 Feiyang is situated over the BL60. It is used to treat hemorrhoids. helps strengthen the kidneys.

BL59 Fuyang - It's located within the Achilles tendon. It enhances its function in the dorsal area.

The BL60 Kunlun located at the top of your feet and is located near your Achilles tendon. The point helps improve movement and strengthens your back.

The BL61 Pucan is about 1.5 cun lower than the BL60. It helps relax the feet, legs and muscles.

The BL62 Shenmai It is located near the foot.

BL63 JinmenThis is on the side that is on the foot.

BL64 Jinggu This is under your feet.

Shugu BL65The Shugu is located beneath the BL65.

The BL66 Tonggu It is one cun from the BL 65 tonggu and is located on the bottom of your pinky.

BL67 Zhiyin is situated in the nail region on the 5th toe (pinky toe).

Kidney

Ki1 Yongquan The location is in the middle in the heel.

The KI2 Rangeu is located at the lower edge of the Navicular bone. This bone is situated on the heel's top.

The KI3 Taixi The location is close to the attachment to the Achilles tendon.

The KI4 Dazhong - This is situated beneath the KI3.

The KI5 Shuiquan is directly beneath the KI4.

KI6 Zhaohai This is situated between KI2 and.

KI7 Fuliu - It's situated over the KI13.

The KI8 Jiaoxin It is situated next to KI8.

KI9 Zhubin - It is located in the lower leg over the feet.

The KI10 Yingu is located on the medial aspect of your knee.

The KI11 Henggu - It can be found in the pelvis.

The KI12 Dahe Dahe is situated just above the KI11.

K13 Qixue K13 Qixue situated 1 cun over K12.

The KI14 Siman - This is one cun higher than KI13.

The KI15 Shuiquan is located one cun over the KI14.

KI16 Huangshu - It is one cup above KI15.

Ki17 Shangou The Shangou is 2 cuns above the navel.

The KI18 Shiguan - This is situated over the KI17.

K19 Yindu It is located just above K18.

Ki20 Futonggu - This is situated over the KI19.

Ki21 Youmen - This is directly above the KI21.

Ki22 Bulang This is located within the breast.

Ki23 Shenfeng - This spot is just above the 22.

Ki24 Lingxu - This location is just above the KI23.

The KI25 Shencang It is an acupuncture spot is situated over the KI24.

Ki26 Yuzhong - It's found in the shoulder region located over the KI25.

Ki27 Shufu The KI27 Shufu is in the shoulder area.

Pericardium

PC1 Tianchi PC1 Tianchi - This acupuncture point is situated near the nupple. It allows chest opening.

PC2 Tianquan - This muscle is situated in between two of the Biceps. It is a perfect match for the heart.

PC3 Quze PC3 Quze - This is situated on the ulnar aspect of the Biceps. It helps to reduce tension and cools the mind.

PC4 Ximen It is located five cuns higher than the wrist's crease. It revigorates blood circulation.

PC5 Jianshi is three cuns higher than the wrist's crease. It's located between carpi flexor as well as the longus of the palmaris.

PC6 Neiguan is located two cuns higher than the wrist's crease. It helps open the chest and enhances the functioning of the digestive system.

PC7 Daling - This is at the center of wristcrease.

PC8 Laogong is located in the middle in the palm.

PC9 Zhongchong is located on the top of your middle finger.

Triple Burner

TB1 Guanchong It is located on the fourth finger.

The TB2 Yemen The TB2 Yemen is situated on the bottom of the 4th finger.

T3 Zhongzhu The Zhongzhu is situated just above the TB2.

The TB4 Yangchi It is located in the wrist region.

The TB5 Waiguan Waiguan is situated over the TB4.

TB6 Zhigou - This is situated above TB5.

The Acupuncture point is situated next to the TB7.

TB8 Sanyangluo This is situated above TB7.

Sidu of TB9 - It is situated over the TB8.

Tianjing TB10 is located 5 cuns above the TB9.

TB11 Qinglengyuan - This is 2 cuns higher than the elbow.

TB12 the Xialuo. This is situated just above TB11.

Naohui TB13 - You can locate this acupuncture point just over the TB12.

The TB14 Janliao is situated in the shoulder region and is above TB13.

The TB15 Tianliao is located in the shoulder blade region.

The TB16 Tianyou It is located on the left from the forehead.

TB17 Yifeng It is located in the lower region of the ear.

Chimai TB18 - This area is behind the ear.

TB19 The Luxi model is situated just above TB19.

TB20 Jiaosun - It is situated on the at the top of the ear.

TB21 Ermen It is located on the top of the head near the ear.

TB22 Erheliao It is located on the left side of the head, close to the ear. It is directly over TB21.

TB23 Sizhukong - It is located near the top of the eyebrow, close to the ear.

Gallbladder

GB1 Tongziliao This is situated just behind the eye.

The GB2 Tinghui point is located on the left of the head. It is near the ear.

GB3 Shanguan - It is located next to GB2.

GB4 Hanyan - This is on the back of the head.

The GB5 Xuanlu file is beneath the GB4.

The GB6 Xuanli can be just beneath the GB5.

The GB7 Qubin is just beneath the GB6.

Shuaigu GB8 - This is located on the left from the top, just above the GB7.

Tianchong, GB9 - This is located next to the GB9.

The GB10 Fubai location is located on the side on the forehead, in the back of the ear.

GB11 Touquiaoyin – This is located beneath GB10.

GB12 Wangu The location is at the back of the head. It is below the ear.

GB13 Benshen. This can be just above the hairline.

GB14 Yangbai The Yangbai GB14 is situated just above the hairline, directly over the eye.

GB15 Linqi - It is situated beside GB13.

The GB16 Muchuang It is at the top on the top of the head.

GB17 Zhengying - It is located one cun over GB16.

GB18 Chengling - This is 1.5 cun higher than the GB17. It's located on at the top.

Naokong GB19 is located to the rear to the front of the head. It is 2.25 cuns away from the GV17.

GB20 Fengchi - This is in the rear side of the head. It is 2.25 cuns away from the GV16.

GB21 Jianjing It is located within trapezius, which is located in your shoulder region. It increases your mobility and also relaxes the tendons.

GB22 Yuanye This is located on the left side of the breast.

GB23 Zhejin It is located below GB23 Zhejin. is the point that is below GB22.

GB24 Riyue - This is located just below the breast.

GB25 Jingmen - It is located near the bottom on the floating rib.

Daimai GB26 This acupuncture is situated beneath the GB25.

GB27 Wushu - It can be found in the abdominal and regulates the uterus as well as the girdling vessel.

GB28 Weidao This acupuncture is located on the right end of stomach.

GBR29 Juliao - This spot is located near the stomach's apex.

GB30 Huantiao The point located in GB30 Huantiao is situated in the buttocks beneath GB29.

GB31 Fengshi located on the bottom of the leg below the GB30.

GB32 Zhongdu - This acupuncture spot is situated on the left side of the leg, just below GB31.

The acupuncture point is located beneath the GB32.

GB34 Yanglingquan - Similar to many gall bladder acupuncture spots, this point is located on one side of your leg. It is situated on one side of knee.

GB35 Yangjiao This is located inside the calf, next to GB36.

GB36 Waiqiu Acupuncture point is located right next to GB35.

The GB37 Guangming Acupuncture spot is located just below the GB36.

GB39 Xuanzhong It is located in the lower leg.

GB40 Qiuxu This acupuncture is situated inside the ankle.

GB41 Zulinqi The point in the vicinity of the pinky's toe.

GB42 Diwuhui - The acupuncture point is situated within the foot, right between head of fourth and fifth metatarsal.

GB43 Xiaxi The Acupuncture point is situated between the fifth between the fifth and fourth toe. It regulates the yang energy in the liver, and also removes excessive body heat and dampness.

GB44 Zuqiaoyin located close to the nail's corner of the fourth toe. It is a brightener for the eyes and regulates the Yang energy of the liver.

Liver

Lv1 Dadun: This point of acupuncture is located on the lateral part of your toe's largest. It's about 0.1 cun away from the point of the toenail's corner.

LV2 Xingjian The LV2 Xingjian location is between the first and second toe. It is the control point for the liver yang, and eliminates the wind in the inside. It soothes the mind, and it eliminates dryness and heat in the body.

LV3 Taichong located on the foot's dorsum, just above the LV2. It regulates the liver yang, relaxes your mind and regulates menstrual flow. It also eases spasms.

LV4 Zhongfeng - This is situated just above LV3 at the ankle.

The LV5 Ligou The Ligou is located five cuns above the ankle. It helps to eliminate the discomfort and warmth within the lower region of the body.

The LV6 Zhongdu - The acupuncture point is located seven cuns above the shinbone. It eliminates obstruction in the channel and relieves abdominal pain.

LV7 Xiguan It is situated near the knee, and is able to relieve the feeling of dampness. It assists in reducing knee pain.

The LV8 Ququan is located on the right side of the knee next to the LV7.

The LV9 Yinbao - This acupuncture spot is located just four cuns over the knee. It regulates the functions in the liver.

The LV10 Zuwuli point is located three cuns below the pubic region. It soothes muscles and ligaments. It also relieves leg pain.

The LV11 Yinlian This Acupuncture point is located just two cuns lower than the pubic region. It relaxes muscles and the tendon. It also aids in relieving leg pain.

The LV12 Jimai The point is located one cun higher than the LV11 point and it's located close to the pubic area within the body.

The LV13 Zhangmen - This location is located on the lateral aspect of the abdomen, below the 11th rib. It enhances the functioning of the spleen and liver. It helps ease rib pain.

The LV14 Qimen is directly below the Nipple. It eliminates stagnation of qi inside the liver. It enhances the functioning of the stomach as well as the liver.

Conception Vessel

CV1 Huiyin is situated within the center of the perineum. It regulates the genitals as well as orifices (nostrils and ear canals the mouth, anus, vagina, nipple and nasolacrimal drains).

CV2 Qugu The CV2 Qugu is located on the upper edge of the pubic region. It improves kidney function and strengthens the functions of the reproductive system.

CV3 Zhongji The location is four cuns to the left of the belly button and over CV2. It helps improve kidney function. It regulates menstrual cycle.

CV4 Guanyuan is located about 2 cun higher than the pubic region. The acupuncture point regulates menstrual flow and also regulates the functioning of the small intestine.

CV5 Shimen The CV5 Shimen is 3 cuns higher than the pubic region. It eliminates dampness in the uterus as well as regulates the qi of the lower portion in the human body.

CV6 Qihai This acupuncture spot is 1.5 cuns far from belly button. It is targeted at the genitals, lower abdomen, and uterus.

CV7 Yinjia0 is located just 1 centimeter below belly button. It regulates the functions of the uterus and menstrual cycle.

CV8 Shenque It is located on in the abdomen button. This acupuncture point helps strengthen the spleen.

CV9 Shuifen - This is approximately 1 cun away from your belly button.

CV10 Xiawan - located two cuns above that belly button.

CV11 Jianli is located three cuns above the CV8 (the stomach button).

CV12 Zhongwan - This acupuncture spot is located just above CV11.

CV13 Shangwan The point lies directly over CV12.

CV14 Juque is situated above CV13.

CV15 Jiuwei - This spot is located seven cuns higher than the belly button. It allows the chest to open and helps with mental problems like obsession, palpation, anxiety, and manic-depressive disorder.

CV16 Zhongting This is situated just below the breasts.

CV17 Tanzhong The Tanzhong is between the nupples. It opens the chest.

CV18 Yutang It is located in the middle of the chest.

CV19 Zigong - This acupuncture point is situated just above CV18.

CV20 Huagai - This acupuncture spot is situated above CV19 and beneath the neck.

CV21 Xuanji: This acupuncture spot is situated between the shoulder blades.

CV22 Tiantu The location is in the neck region.

CV23 Lianquan It is located beneath the jaw.

CV24 Chengjiang located beneath the mouth.

The Governing Vessel

GV1 Changqiang The area is situated between the anus as well as the coccyx. This point is used to treat manic-depression, epilepsy, and hemorrhoids.

It is GV2 Yaoshu It is in the area of the anus and helps strengthen the lower back.

GV3 Yaoyangguan - This is located at on the L4. It helps strengthen the legs and lower back.

The GV4 Mingmen It is situated in the rear, between L3 and.

The GV5 Xuanshu point is located in low back just over GV4.

GV6 JizhongThe Jizhong is located behind, just below T11. It helps improve the functioning of the spleen. It also eliminates internal wind.

The GV7 Zhongshu - This point helps strengthen the spine as well as the spleen.

The GV8 Jinsuo area is situated beneath T9 and helps to relax the tendons.

It is also known as GV9 Zhiyang The acupuncture point is located below on the back of your upper. This point controls the gallbladder as well as the liver. It also opens the chest.

GV10 Lingtai - This lies in the lower back, above the GV9. It is a source of heat that can be removed.

It is a GV11 Shendao It is situated in the back, just above the neck. It assists in removing the hot air in the lung.

The GV12 Shenzhu The GV12 Shenzhu is situated in the midline area, near the top of the back. It reduces the heat in the lung and eliminates internal wind.

GV13 Taodao - This acupuncture spot is in the back, just beneath the neck.

The GV14 Dazhui is located in the back of neck. It assists in easing fatigue.

The GV15 Yamen is located in the rear at the top.

The GV16 Fengfu - This is the point that lies in the middle in the head.

GV17 Naohu - This acupuncture spot is situated just above the head, and it is able to snuff out the inner wind.

GV18 Qiangjian is just above G17 at the middle in the neck. It helps to calm the mind and eliminates internal wind.

Houding, GV19 - This is located in the middle in the front.

GV20 Baihui - This acupuncture spot is just above the head, and between the ears.

GV21 Qianding – This acupuncture point is located above the head, above GV20.

GV22 Xinhui This is 1.5 cuns higher than GV21. it assists in reducing mental anxiety as well as stress athletes commonly encounter.

The GV23 Shangxing is situated in the middle on the top of your head. It lifts the nose and brightens the eyes.

Shenting GV24 - This is situated directly above the hairline and in the middle of the hairline.

Acupuncture GV25 Suliao points is located near the top on the nasal bridge. It helps relieve rhinitis.

GV26 Renzhong - This is situated in between the lip of your lower and the nose.

GV27 Diuduan This is situated near the top of the upper lip.

The GV28 Yianjiao The Yianjiao GV28 is near the gums.

Extra

EX1 Sishencong EX1 Sishencong Sishencong has four points on in the upper part of the head. It is just one cun from GV20.

EX2 Yintang It is located the area between your eyes. It eliminates the wind in your head and soothes the mind.

EX3 Taiyang Acupuncture point EX3 Taiyang is located near the top of your eyebrow. It is responsible for the functioning of the liver and helps improve your eyesight.

EX4 Yuyao is located in between the eyebrows. It regulates the function in the liver.

EX5 Bitong-This acupuncture spot is located on the left right side of the nose. It is able to open the nose and helps treat nasal inflammation.

EX6 Jingzhong is located in the hips, next to CV6.

EX7 Qimen - It is situated below EX6.

EX8 Zigong The location is on the sacral part of the.

EX9 Tituo – This is located 4 cuns in the lateral direction of CV4.

EX10 Dingchuan EX10 Dingchuan Dingchuan is situated at the back of the neck, just beside the GV14. It helps improve the function of the lungs , and helps to reduce breathlessness.

EX11 Jinggong The EX11 Jinggong is located on the right side of the stomach, and next to the BL52.

EX12 Huatuojiaji It is located approximately 0.5 cuns to the spinal column. This acupuncture spot strengthens spinal column.

EX13 Shiquihuixia. This is located at the bottom of the spine. It improves the lower back.

EX14 Jianneiling - It is located close to the armpits, and is below LI15.

EX15 Baxie It is found within five fingers that are webbed. It loosens the tendons in fingers, wrists, and hands.

EX16 Shixuan It is located near the end of your finger.

EX17 Xiyan It is located inside the knee. It eliminates wind.

EX18 Dannangxue The location is on the knee's side and can cause discomfort.

EX19 Laweixue is located on the upper end on the bottom leg the middle between ST36 as well as ST37.

EX20 Bafeng - It is found inside the infra-red of toes. It loosens the tendons and helps reduce stiffness and spasms of the foot.

EX21 Erjian The EX21 Erjian is situated at the back of the ear.

EX22 Anmian EX22 Anmian located in the navel area.

EX23 Qipang The acupuncture point EX23 Qipang is located just above the wrist.

EX24 Erbai The EX24 Erbai situated in the middle of your hand. It is used to treat neck pain.

EX25 Luozhen EX25 Luozhen situated in the middle of the hand between the middle finger and index finger.

EX26 Yaotongxue EX26 Yaotongxue Yaotongxue is made up of two points situated between the fifth finger and fourth finger, and between index and middle finger. These points assist in treating lower back pain as well as improve mobility.

EX27 Heding spot is situated just above the knee and can treat knee injuries.

EX28 Neimadian EX28 Neimadian found on the medial leg. It helps with leg pain and inflammation following surgery.

EX29 Naoqing EX29 Naoqing situated right above your ankle. It helps with cognitive confusion and enhances functioning.

For certain sports injuries there is a need to apply the acupuncture points when performing the cupping procedure. In other instances it is possible to utilize trigger points.

Chapter 9: Common Sports Injuries And How

To Use Sports Cupping To Treat These

Injuries to your body do not only impact how you perform, however, it may be extremely harmful to impact to your overall health. Some sports injuries have severe psychological consequences.

Here's a list with the most frequently occurring sports injuries, and the best way to use cupping therapy to cure these.

Ankle injuries

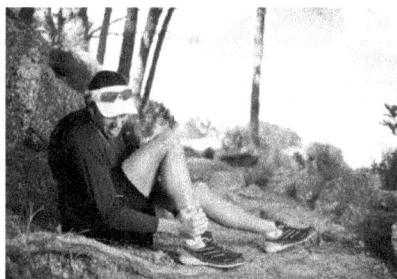

Many athletes make use of sports cupping to relieve ankle injuries. Ankle injuries can be difficult to heal and can impact mobility. The swelling and bruising that is associated with an ankle injury may result in a sprain.

Footballers, surfers triathletes, snowboarders players, karate players and cricketers are prone to injuries to the ankle. To treat this issue, you can employ a the medium-to-strong cupping technique for the area that has been injured after the swelling has diminished. It is also possible to apply cups on points of acupuncture, such as SP5 Shangqui and BL60 Kulun, BL62 Shenmai K8, Jiaoxin and the K3 Taixi. You could also use the Hijama cupping technique on BL-62 or ST-41 Jiexi.

Achilles Tendonitis

It is the Achilles tendon forms the strong tendon that connects your heel with the muscles of the calf. It is also referred to by the name of the calcaneal tendon. It lets you walk and allows you to stand on the tip of your toes. It is the strongest and biggest tendon that exists in your body. It is located directly below the skin. It doesn't have any kind of protective cover, which means it is more prone to injury and inflammation.

Achilles tendonitis can affect basketball players, squash players, divers, triathletes, pro-level dancers and rugby athletes and soccer players. It is result of overtraining, an abrupt intensification of exercise, additional bone growth and tight muscles of the calf. The symptoms of this disorder are discomfort and stiffness along the Achilles tendon. If you're suffering from this disorder you'll experience discomfort and swelling on your feet following exercise. Achilles tendonitis happens to be one of the most commonly reported sports injuries. In reality, it is responsible for 5-10% of all athletic injuries.

To treat this issue to treat this condition, you can use this moving cupping (massage cupping) technique on the Achilles tendon starting at the acupuncture spot the BL57 Chengjin up to the calcaneus. Be sure to obtain a consent from your doctor prior to doing this procedure.

Achilles Tendon Rupture

It is a total tears of Achilles tendon. This is a problem for rugby players who jump cyclists, runners and gymnasts as well as volleyball players, football players, as well as tennis players. People who have this disorder experience an intense pain in the Achilles tendon. The use of cups is not recommended.

Medial Tibial Stress Syndrome

The medial Tibial Stress Syndrome is a condition that occurs on an area on the outside of your outside leg. It is often referred to in the form of Shin Splints. This condition is caused by repeated trauma to connective tissue that surrounds Shin bone (tibia). The weak core muscles, the inflexibility or tight leg and muscle imbalances can increase the risk of developing of this disorder.

Shin splints are a problem for athletes participating in the sports of running and endurance running. It is a problem for tennis players, squash athletes, footballers gymnasts, triathletes, runners and basketball players as well as volleyball players.

To treat this problem To treat this disorder, apply cupping therapy on the outer portion of the bone that runs along the side. Place the cupping cup upon ST36 Zusanli before moving it towards ST39 Xiajuxu. Repeat the process two times a week for at minimum two weeks.

Knee Injury

It is also the largest and most massive joint. It is enclosed by the synovial capsule, which is a sac filled with fluid. synovial capsule. This capsule connects your lower leg with the leg that is higher. The overuse and trauma of the leg may cause knee injuries. The condition can affect athletes, runners basketball players, high jumpers, rugby players and golfers. and martial artists.

To treat knee injuries You can do medium cupping ST35 Dubi and the GB34 Yanglingquan Liv8 Quguan Heiding Extra as well as ST34 Liangqui. It is also possible to apply Hijama cupping to the spot of the injury.

Iliotibial Band Syndrome

This is among the most frequent injuries from overuse in athletes. It's characterised by pain and aching on the lateral part of the knee and hip. It's usually caused by irritation between hip bones and the iliotibial band. The athletes who suffer from this condition have a burning, sharp sensation in the hip and knee.

Iliotibial band syndrome is a problem for triathletes, cyclists and runners soccer players, weightlifters, tennis players and squash players.

To alleviate this, perform a the medium and strong cupping technique on the lateral aspect of your knee. It is also possible to shift the cup towards the Tensor Fascia. It is also possible to put cups to the GB30 Huantiao.

Hamstring Injuries

Hamstring injuries may limit mobility and can take longer to heal. For athletes who have injuries to their hamstrings, it is advised to rest for a couple of weeks.

This injury is affecting football, rugby as well as cricketers. To treat it, you must perform a cupping from the BL36 Chengfu up to BL40 Weizhong. If the problem is rooted in the back of the spine it is also necessary to cup DU3 Yaoyanoggguan and BL28 Pangguang along with BL26 Guanyuanshu.

Quadriceps Femoris Injuries

The quadriceps, also known as quadriceps femoris is located on just in front of your thigh. It is composed of four parts: vastus medialis, vastuslateralis as well as the vastus intermedius and the rectus femoris. The injury is common among athletes, including those who play rugby and football.

To treat this issue Apply a the medium and light cupping technique on the outer part of your quadriceps (vastus lateralis) and then move towards the front of your quadriceps muscles femoris (rectus Femoris).

The hip and the groin are both painful.

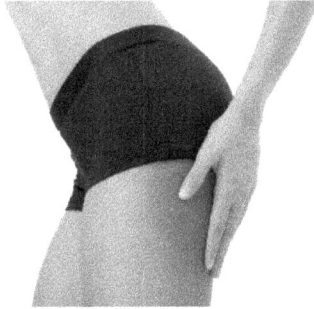

The area houses a variety of vital organs like the small intestinal tract, the ureter and cecum and the colon that ascends the large intestinal tract, fallopian tube and an ovary. If you feel discomfort in this region be sure to consider it a serious issue. It also houses a number of ligaments, tendons veins, arteries, bone structures and nerves. The groin and hip area is also where you can put a lot of the weight of performing household chores or engaging in sports activities.

The hip is essentially the socket and ball joint that connects your pelvis and femur. There are a variety of sports like walking, running and jumping can affect the hip. The wrong footwear and the numbness to the back of lower muscles may cause hip discomfort. The majority of hip pain is due to injuries from contact sports, such as ruptures, contusions, or ligament injuries.

Basketball, golf as well as footballers are prone to groin and hip discomfort because they tend to twist their bodies frequently.

To treat hip pain, use the medium cupping technique to lower back muscles, such as the BL-53 Baohuang, the BL-28 Panngu and the GB-30 Huantiao.

To relieve groin pain, utilize the cupping method that moves starting at the BL 28 Pangguangshu and shift the cup to GB28.

Buttock Pain

The athletes who are involved in sprinting or football often suffer from buttock discomfort. The pain could be confined in the buttocks or it could be associated with posterior thigh discomfort or the lower back. The majority of this pain is due to problems with the sacroiliac joint, spinal lumbar region, and the hamstring attachments to the bony portions of the butt, also known as ischial tuberosities. But, in some cases, buttock pain is caused by more serious health conditions such as ankylosing spondylitis, spondyloarthropathies, psoriatic arthritis, Reiter's syndrome, malignancy, and arthritis associated with inflammatory bowel disease.

Buttock pain may limit your movements and negatively impact your performance. To relieve the localized pain in your buttock (meaning that you feel only pain in the area of your buttock) apply a the medium-to-strong cupping technique on EM-Yaoyan. Also, the BL54 Zhibian and the GB30 Huantiao and the BL28 Pangguangshu.

If you feel any discomfort in your legs as well as lower back muscles, you can try the cupping method of moving by following the direction of your gluteus maxus muscle.

Lower Back Injuries

The pain of the back in lower backs is among the most frequently reported medical conditions in the sports and general population. Many athletes suffer lower back pain due to the tension or tightness in the muscles of the lower back.

The tight or stretched lower back muscles can cause spasms, which can limit circulation of blood in the muscles. This could limit your movement and adversely affect how you perform in your sport. There are many causes that can cause lower back pain. These include:

Twisting the spine and lifting

* Lifting heavy objects

* Bad posture

* Excessive use of the Lumbar spine

The repetitive swinging movements required for basketball, tennis golf, squash, cricket and racquetball could cause irritation and damage to the vertebrae, ligaments and discs in the spinal column. Stress fractures in the spine that occur in contact sports may result in chronic discomfort and limit your movement.

Golfers as well as runners and tennis players are at risk of low back pain. If the pain is confined to the lower back, use cupping to GV3 Yaoyangguan, the BL28 Pangguangshu and the BL26 Guanyuanshu.

If your lower back pain is located in the lower back area, however, it is radiating towards buttocks, put the cups on GV3 Yaoyangguan, the BL54 Zhibian and the BL53 Baohuang. Utilize cupping that is light to moderate. Allow the cups to rest in the skin 15 minutes.

In case your back has become stiff you could apply the cupping treatment by following the path of the muscle affected. For instance, when you treat the stiff erector spinae muscles your cupping movements should follow the direction through the muscle. That means you must move the cup with a vertical movement. It is recommended to perform the therapy at least twice each week for a period of five weeks. It typically takes between ten and twenty cupping sessions to reduce lower back pain.

Shoulder Injuries

Shoulder injuries are the 2nd most frequently reported complaint by athletes, following back pain. The shoulder is among the most difficult body parts to treat. The shoulder can be described as a complicated joint, which is connected via ligaments and straps like muscles referred to as "rotator cuffs". The shoulder is composed of three bones: the scapula, the clavicle as well as the humerus. It also consists of four joints, which are:

The GH (Glenohumeral) Joint The GH (Glenohumeral) Joint and socket joint which connects with the upper arm (humerus) with the scapula (shoulder blade).

SC (Sternoclavicular) Joint The joint is between the clavicle as well as the sternum.

AC (Acromioclavicular) Joint The AC joint is located situated between the clavicle (collarbone) and the top portion of your shoulder blade referred to as the acromion.

St. (Scapulothoracic) Joint The joint is located between the rib cage and scapula.

Athletics who play throwing sports like baseball, rugby golf, hockey, volleyball, tennis as well as Australian football are at risk of shoulder injuries. Weight lifters, gymnasts, swimmers, cyclists and shot-putters too suffer from these kinds of injuries at times. About 40% of athletes suffering from shoulder-related injuries experience AC joint injuries.

These are some of the more frequent kinds that shoulder pain can be:

Adhesive Capsulitis , Frozen Shoulder or Frozen Should

Active athletes are not prone to injury. However, it's an extremely serious problem that is affecting older athletes. It is caused by the irritation or excessive use of the GH joint. It can also be due to various ailments like breast surgery, diabetes, trauma, and hypothyroidism. If you are suffering from this disorder your shoulder movements are restricted and painful.

Acromioclavicular Joint Arthrosis or AC Joint Degeneration

The reason for this is the overuse by this AC joint. If you suffer from this condition you may experience discomfort in the front in your shoulder. The pain could extend to your neck, arm, or the chest.

Ailment to the Rotator Cuff

Rotator cuffs are small , but robust muscles that surround the shoulder. There are four kinds of rotator muscles, which are the subscapularis teres minor and supraspinatus. They are also known as infraspinat. The teres minor as well as the infraspinatus muscle are external rotators. The subscapularis is an internal muscle that flexes the glenohumeral (GH) joint. If you raise your arms excessively you could be prone to injuries to your rotator-cuff.

For treating shoulder injuries, it is recommended to use four pieces of the size 2 or 3 cups. Apply a medium cupping technique to your TCM (traditional Chinese medicine) areas that are near the shoulder joint, specifically LI2 Yunmen SI9 Jianzhen SP20 Zhouron SI10 Naoshu SI11 Tianzhong SJ14 Jianliao as well as LI16 Jugu. If you also feel pain in your arm, you can add LI14Binao, Li15 Jianyu and SJ13 Naohui. If you also feel pain in your neck, you could include cups on SI12 Bingfeng as well as SJ15 Tianlao. SJ15 is situated within GB21 Jianjing along with SI13 Quyuan. Allow the cups to sit for 10 to 20 minutes, based on the extent that the injury has.

It is possible to use the moving cupping therapy for all kinds shoulders injuries. However, you should avoid using this technique on injuries to the shoulder that are dislocated. Be sure to follow the direction that the muscles of your shoulder follow while lifting the cup. It is also recommended to combine cupping and acupuncture therapy to treat shoulder injuries.

Insomniac Syndrome

Training can cause some loss of energy and performance. This is known as Underperformance Syndrome. According to an issue of Sports Injury Bulletin published in 2002, UUPS or Unexplained Underperformance Syndrome is the term used to describe a pattern of fatigue and diminished performance that is not due to a medical reason and even after 2 months of rest. This condition was identified at the end of 1999 by an team of researchers from Oxford University. The condition affects 2 percent to 10 percent of endurance athletes with elite performance. The most frequent manifestation of this condition.

In the competitive world of sports, coaches tend to intensify the training when an athlete is not performing. This increases fatigue and reduces performance.

Before using the cupping treatment to treat this disorder, you should apply the tongue diagnostic technique that is part of conventional Chinese medicine to identify the root causes of the syndrome of underperformance. To determine this, take a examine the tongue of the patient and look at the colour.

Blood Injury

It sounds hilarious. How can the blood be damaged? It is a liquid that's transformed from the substance of the water and food you consume. It is made by the activity of the Qi. It circulates through the body and feeds tissues of the body. It is a source of energy or qi. Qi circulates wherever blood flows. A blood injury occurs in the event that your body has been exhausted or you are consuming an unhealthy diet. It can also be result of other factors like an excessive amount of sexual activity, continuous bleeding, or an intense workout routine. When your blood has been damaged you'll feel dizzy and insomnia, as well as heart palpitations, aching bones and muscles. It's also possible to be unable to breathe and sweating profusely.

To alleviate qi and blood stagnation, blood circulation has to be improved. It is possible to do this through placing the cup in the front of your chest for around 15 minutes each day. It is also possible to place cups on the LU1 Zhongfu and the LU2 Yunmen as well as the entire back.

Forearm and Elbow Injury

Athletes are prone to elbow and forearm injuries which can affect joints, muscles bones, ligaments, bony joints, tendon and nerves. The cause is the overtraining process or a collision on the field. If the injury was result of an on-field collision, avoid cupping therapy. The patient should be transported to the hospital as soon as possible. Cupping therapy is the only therapy for forearm and elbow injuries that result from excessive use or overtraining.

Athletes who are involved in swimming, golf basketball, racquet sport, bowling, baseball ski, weightlifting, rock climbing, gymnastics or kayaking can be more vulnerable to elbow and forearm injuries.

To treat forearm and elbow injuries, use either stationary or moving cupping therapies to the area affected.

Be aware that cupping therapy for sports injuries that are commonplace should be performed by licensed Therapists.

Chapter 10: Everything You Need To Learn

About The Bruises

The suction generated through the cup will likely leave marks upon the surface. Butdon't be concerned this is only temporary.

However, there's a important thing you should be aware of about the marks. The texture and color of the cup marks could be a good indicator of the health of your body.

Bright Red Cupping Marks

This means that there's an excessive amount of heat in the area and there could be inflammation. In this case it's important to utilize the technique of flash cupping because the skin might leak. You must apply cooling balms to treat the spots. However, you should not make use of the ice.

Purple Blue

If the skin appears to be purple blue after cupping, this means that there is stagnation. This means that the winds are stuck in the region and is unable to move. This is known as "lamig" within the Philippines. It is possible to use heating therapy to disperse the winds in the area. If you're experiencing stagnation in a particular area in your body it's recommended to massage that area frequently.

Dark Blue to Purple Black

If the skin's color ranges from dark blue or black, that means there is a build-up of toxic substances within this region. This also indicates it's "poison wind" in the area. The blood flowing through that region in your body has become toxic , and it must be eliminated.

Pale Bluish

If the skin appears light white after cupping, it's because there isn't enough blood flow in the area due to energy obstruction. If this occurs then stop cupping and apply heat or a hot balm on the region.

Deep Red to Magenta

This is a sign that there's stagnant heat within the region. The skin might be bleeding. After cupping, you may use a trauma liniment. It can reduce swelling and help soothe your skin.

Dark Gray

If your skin appears darker gray following the cupping was removed, it means the toxins are re-settling in the body. It is necessary to flush out the toxins by cupping that area once more or applying balms.

If the marks from cupping are not gone after 2 weeks, it is time to visit an Therapist. You might also have to see a dermatologist if you have significant skin damage.

Chapter 11: Of Frequently Asked Questions

Concerning Cupping

Here's a list with frequently asked questions regarding cupping therapy.

1. Are cupping cups risk-free?

Yes. The methods within this publication are secure and efficient when applied by a qualified professional.

2. Can I perform this treatment on myself?

Yes, you can perform cupping to the front of your physique. If you're not experienced, you should employ an expert. If you try this yourself, it will not bring the results you desire particularly for certain illnesses however it could be efficient for relaxation.

3. Do I have to be concerned about marks following cupping?

Yes, marks are inevitable. However, they will fade in two days and one week, at the most. The duration of healing typically is dependent on the intensity of the treatment as well as the long the cups remained over the face.

4. Does it cause pain?

The majority of the time it won't. There will be a pulsing sensation. In some instances intense cupping could cause discomfort that is a sign that the pressure must be raised to more manageable levels.

5. Does cupping cause skin damage?

Not at all. The marks you'll notice after cupping are only temporary. The reddish spots are a sign that there's a higher circulation of blood in the area of your body.

6. Do I have to cup my face?

Yes, but you must use the gentle cupping technique for your face. It is also necessary to utilize the smaller cup (cup no. 4 5, 6, and 4)

7. Do I have the right to cup the inside of my bodily parts?

It's not a problem, but it could cause issues.

8. Do I feel tired following my cupping treatment?

It's likely that you'll be a bit weaker following the cupping session. However, some are energized after the cupping treatment.

9. Do cupping therapies have any negative side consequences?

Yes. Apart from the marks that appear to your face, you may also experience intense hunger following the treatment. There could be sleepiness, vivid dreams nausea, headaches, and chills. There is a possibility of having a the body smell to be strong due to the detox.

10. How many times will I need to undergo cupping before I be able to see the results?

It depends. You can notice improvements after just one or two sessions of cupping therapy.

11. Do you have the ability to use cupping therapy for cancer patients?

Yes, you can. It's a powerful treatment for pain in cancer patients. However, the energy level and the general health of the patient have to be considered prior to conducting the session.

12. Where can I go to receive cupping therapy?

You can go to TCM (traditional Chinese medicine) clinics. Many coaches for sports, Olympic trainers, and physical therapists also perform cupping therapy.

13. You can use cupping therapy to complement your treatment?

Yes. Cupping therapy is a viable option in conjunction with traditional medical treatments. However, if you're taking high doses medication, you should discuss the possibility of cupping with your doctor.

14. Do I have to do cupping therapy if I'm suffering from an illness that causes fever?

No. Don't try cupping in case you are suffering from hyperthermia or you're overly exuberant.

15. Are you able to do cupping therapy with a full stomach?

Avoid cupping therapy if you are hungry, to avoid fainting or weakness that is severe. Take a bite of food a of food prior to doing the treatment.

16. Are cupping therapies suitable for children as well as for older people?

Generally, yes. However, you are able to employ a light cupping method, and you need to take it very seriously.

17. Why am I seeing bruises?

The suction produced by the cup is able to draw out old, stagnant, and un-circulating blood from the region, and brings it on the outside of your skin. The result can be a mark called "sha'.

18. How long will each session last?

Massage is a common practice for therapists also, and a session can last from 30 or more minutes up to one hour. The cupping process itself could last between 10 and 15 minutes in the initial session.

19. What can I do following the treatment?

It is essential to drink plenty of fluids to flush out all of the toxic substances that were drained out. Be sure to take enough rest following the procedure, and don't perform any strenuous physical exercise. Famous and professional athletes are not afraid to show the marks of cupping. However, in order to prevent infection ensure that all marks are properly covered. Also, avoid drinking alcohol on the day of the procedure.

20. Are they expensive?

A lot of people believe that cupping therapy is costly because it's the latest trend in fashion, but it's actually fairly inexpensive. According to 2017 data, each session is priced between $40 and the range of $80 to $40.

Cupping for sports isn't so popular as traditional treatment, however several studies suggest that it could dramatically improve the performance of athletes. So why do sports stars such as Michael Phelps believe in it.

Chapter 12: What Exactly Is Cupping?

Cupping therapy is a long-standing alternative form of medicine that has been practiced since around 1500 B.C., over 3,500 years in the past. It was first mentioned in Egyptian hieroglyphics and is referred to out as a"great medicine" as part of the Quran. Cupping has been utilized in Chinese medicine since the fourth or third century A.D. and is still frequently used in traditional Chinese medicine as well as at the modern Chinese hospitals. But its popularity has increased dramatically in recent times. In the process, it's becoming more readily accessible in the fields of sports medicine, Acupuncture, therapeutic massage and alternative medical centers across Europe, the U.S., Asia, and Europe.

Cupping is the process of using suction cups typically made of silicone or glass on the body in order to create an inverse pressure over the area being treated. This draws blood to the skin's surface. Cupping can cause the appearance of bruises on the skin. They appear like the appearance of a Hickey. These recognizable marks were popularized through American swimming star Michael Phelps, an avid advocate of cupping therapy in the Olympic Games in 2016. Olympics held in Rio De Janeiro.

The size and the number of cups used will depend on the type of treatment being used, but when performed by a certified practitioner, cupping therapy can be utilized to treat many ailments. It can be applied practically everywhere in the human body. This includes feet and the face.

Based on Dr. Houman Danesh, a pain treatment specialist in the Mount Sinai Hospital in New York Cupping can help jumpstart our body's own healing by improving the flow of blood in the area of treatment. It's a way of improving the healing process as well as soothing painful joints and muscles.

Cupping was done using natural materials such as animal horns bamboo tubes ceramic vessels, hollowed-out the bones of coconut, coconut hulls gourds and seashells. Cupping treatments used in the early days included drawing out poison of bites from animals or insects and removing fluids from wounds or skin lesions. In certain ancient cultures, healers also utilized cupping to aid in drawing out evil spirits.

Cupping therapy in the present is generally carried out using silicone or glass cups, however bamboo tubes, and even horns have been employed in certain parts in the entire world. Fire cupping traditionally is done by heating the interior of the cup using alcohol, a flammable liquid, or a similar combustible substance such as herbs, after which placing the cup in the warm position on the skin of the area being treated. As the cup cools the amount of air within the cup decreases, causing suction within the cup. Nowadays, many professionals make use of cups that have valves that are coupled to an electric hand pump or similar device to produce suction.

It has been demonstrated that cups bring a myriad of positive health effects , such as improving lymphatic circulation and blood flow as well as pain management, decreasing inflammation, healing of injuries sustained in sports, improving feelings of mental relaxation and wellbeing, as well as being an example of deeply tissue massage. Cupping can also assist patients relax and create a feeling of physical and mental peace. Additionally, since it can help soothe nerves, the cupping method offers potential for treating anxiety, stress, and various mental illnesses.

Chapter 13: Different Types Of Cupping

There are three methods to cupping. They are dry, massage cupping, as well as wet. In both dry and wet cupping, therapists will place a substance that is flammable like alcohol, herbs or paper in glass cups and ignite it. When the fire has gone out and the cup is set with its open end towards the skin of the patient. As the air inside of the cup cools, it reduces in size and creates the impression of a vacuum. This results in the skin as well as the underlying tissues to expand and become redder as blood vessels increase. The cup is placed in the cup for anywhere between 3 and 10 minutes, based on the type of cupping. Certain modern cupping methods utilize a pump made of rubber instead of heating to create the vacuum within the cup.

Based on your requirements and the location they are applied to your body at throughout the treatment, the practitioner will use between three to six cups and possibly up to 10. For the first session, your Therapist will typically start using just two or three cups, or perhaps one cup to determine what happens.

Dry Cupping

Dry cupping is the most usual form of treatment. It involves the therapist placing a number of glass cups or bulbs onto the skin of the patient at certain locations along the body. The cups are then placed under a vacuum through the application of heat, and removal of heat, or by the application of a small, portable pump connected on the vessels.

In an uninvolved cupping session the vessel or glass is heated by the use of a substance that is flammable, such as alcohol. After the cup has been warm, the practitioner will place the cups on top of the skin. The cup's temperature decreases as the air inside is shrinking, creating the impression of a vacuum. This makes the cup stick on the skin. The negative pressure in the cup can cause the skin and the surrounding tissues to rise up into the mouth of the glass. The pressure creates blood to flow to the area being treated, which causes the skin to begin to redden. Typically, the glasses or silicone cups are positioned for three to ten minutes However, certain treatments require longer time and may last for up to 20 minutes.

Dry cupping causes a minimal amount of pressure . It is ideal for use on soft tissue which creates a secure and tightly bonded seal to the skin. Cupping can cause redness to the skin, and a bit of swelling in the area of treatment due to blood and bodily fluids which accumulate beneath the skin. However, it doesn't usually cause any major degree of discomfort. For most patients, the discomfort is usually the sensation of a small pinch in the course of treatment, and then a feeling of relaxation after removal of the cups. Sometimes, minor blisters could occur, but the healer will explain that it is a sign that the treatment was efficient in targeting the affected area of the body.

Massage Cupping

Massage cupping is one type of dry cupping which uses silicon cups rather than glass that are able to be moved over the skin of the patient for an effect similar to massage. Myofascial decompression is the method of using movements of range during your massage session.

The practice of massage cupping is also referred to as Ventosa cupping is a type of massage therapy that involves the practitioner shifts the cups during the session, moving them over your skin and all over your body. In a sense, cupping is an alternative to traditional massage therapy. Instead of exerting pressure downwards on the area of treatment massage cupping employs suction that pulls the skin muscles, and tissues up away from your body's center. It's an ancient method that has been utilized for centuries as a method of healing in a variety of different cultures, including traditional Chinese treatment for many illnesses. Nowadays, massage cupping is considered to be an efficient, non-invasive, and inexpensive alternative treatment that can be utilized as a stand-alone treatment or with other therapies.

In a cupping massage, the therapist carries cup back and forth across the muscle fibers to break up adhesions and reduce scarring on the fascial and muscular tissue. Cupping massage has been found to increase circulation, improve lung capacity and endurance and aid in detoxification by improving lymphatic drainage. Apart from its application in healing injuries massage cupping is also used to maintain the body and as a pre-event injury prevention treatment.

Like other types of cupping, the massage therapy employs downward pressure that pulls the skin muscles, connective tissue upwards to improve circulation and encourage healing. Massage cupping is utilized for physical therapy as an addition to chiropractic treatments as well as offered as a spa treatment. Massage cupping has proven beneficial for various ailments such as the management of pain, stress relief and relaxation of the mind and muscles as well as weight loss and for sleep aids and as a treatment for cellulite.

Massage cupping practitioners typically utilize silicone therapy cups since they are soft and flexible, making it simpler as well as more relaxing for the therapist to move the cups over the client's body. Before placing the cups, the body of the patient is covered with a large amount of oil in order to ensure the proper lubrication needed for the cups to glide smoothly across the skin. The suction and pressure generated by massage cupping release the stiff tissue, breaks down and eliminates any excessive fluids and toxins. dissolves adhesions and stimulates connective tissue and increases the circulation of lymphatic and blood fluids in stagnant areas of the muscles and the skin.

Myofascial Decompression Cupping

Myofascial decompression is an alternative to massage cupping, which also includes movements of range of motion during your cupping sessions. This kind of massage therapy can be beneficial in regards to breaking down scar tissue and opening adhesions from the fascia that may result from injuries sustained in sports or damage to tissues from other traumas.

Fascia is the tightly woven material of connective tissue that divides the body, covers, and stabilizes muscles, ligaments, tendons as well as other soft tissues throughout the body. It's not just the lining that protects and separates various tissues, including ligaments, muscles, as well as organs. The fascia is also an unbroken structure that runs through every part of your body much like the yarn in the sweater, although the arms are distinct from body part of the garment as is the fiber continuous and found throughout the entire garment creating structure and connecting all the parts into one.

The fascia is made up primarily of collagen, and is comparable in composition to ligaments as well as tendon. It also provides structural support, some of the main roles of the fascia is less friction due to the use of force that allows muscles to move smoothly across one another. Furthermore, fascia is also a moving wraparound for blood vessels and nerves when they travel through and between muscles. The fascia tissue can be classified into three main components:

Superficial fascia is the skin's lowermost layer skin (dermis) serves as a storage space for water and fat, and also serves as a pathway for blood vessels and nerves and blood vessels

Visceral fascia: membranes that help support, suspend and wrap around the organs in the body cavity

* Deep fascia The dense connective tissue of fibrous fibers that penetrates and covers the soft tissue that is associated to the system of skeletal. This includes the ligaments, muscles bones, and tendons.

In a healthy, normal state the fascia is at ease and able for stretching and moving freely without limitation. But, if the body is subjected to physical injuries or inflammation, scarring as well as emotional or physical traumas, the fascia can be unable to stretch and may become restrictive or tight. The loss of flexibility in the fascia could be the result of injury like a fall whiplash, or car accident surgery, or the result of repeated strain injuries.

In time, the fascial tightening may cause a buildup in tension and pressure on the body's rest because of diminished blood flow and accumulation of toxic substances. If untreated for a long time and this causes the fascia to become stiff and lose its flexibility, which can cause pain in the affected area. Since fascia is a robust, extremely connected web of tissue, an accumulation of tension in one area can cause an effect that ripples across the entire body, or, in certain instances, a shadow effect in which an issue in one area of the body manifests as discomfort in the other. This is why we could be experiencing pain in our knee or thigh which does not have anything to do with an injury to the leg or knee however it is because of a problem in the lower back.

The term "myofascial" refers to treating simultaneously muscles ("myo") and fascia throughout a single therapy procedure. Myofascial release, also known as decompression therapy is a method that uses gentle pressure on connective tissue, allowing it to stretch, thereby reducing pain and restoring range motion.

Myofascial Decompression Cupping is the practice of incorporating myofascial compression therapy as a part of an hour-long massage cupping session. In practice this implies that exercises in range of motion are done in conjunction alongside the deeper tissue massage elements in massage cupping. The mix of pressure created by the cups and the range of motion exercises help release adhesions and reduce scarring of connective tissue, allowing the body to return to function prior to injury.

Wet Cupping

Wet cupping is based on the same principles of dry cupping, however it is a step more advanced by using a series of small cuts or perforations within the skin in order to stimulate circulation of tiny amount of blood through the vessel. The idea of the practice is that harmful substances as well as other harmful substances found in the blood are drawn into the area of treatment through negative pressure. By drawing blood out of the body causes elimination of these unhealthy substances in the human body. It aids in healing.

Wet cupping is a method of bloodletting that is utilized to eliminate stagnant blood, remove body heat, as well as to relieve pain. Cupping with wet, often referred to as hijama is an old therapy practice with Islamic origin. In Arabic the word hijama translates to "to suckle" in order to "return to a state" of inner balance. It was deemed to be the "best of all medicines" which was highly supported by Prophet Muhammad and specifically mentioned in the Quran for its numerous health advantages. Wet cupping remains well-known across several Muslim countries around the world.

Wet cupping is an all-encompassing treatment method that assists in returning the body back to a healthy alkaline state by neutralizing acidity and increasing the process of removing stagnant blood. This leads to the elimination of harmful elements and toxins from the body. This helps it regenerate and heal its own body.

Wet cupping -- also known as medicinal bleeding uses a gentler suction technique than other types of cupping. It's done through a multi-step procedure. The procedure begins with a brief period of dry cupping that is used to draw blood into the area of treatment. The therapist then takes out the cups, scrapes or creates small cuts into the skin that has been raised in the area being treated. The traditional Chinese cupping, the cuts are made using three-pronged needles. Modern Western methods typically employ scalpels or lancets. Contrary to this, Islamic hijama cupping propagates blood flow through scraping the skin. After this procedure is completed, the therapist puts the cups in the same position that they were in for the cupping process and uses suction, which draws out a tiny amount of blood. Wet cupping advocates believe that the removal of this blood leads to the removal of harmful substances and toxic substances from the body, which aids in healing. But this claim has not yet been confirmed scientifically.

It is crucial to clean the skin and sterilized before and after a cupping treatment to avoid infections to the cupping sites. In some instances, you might receive an antibiotic ointment or bandsages to limit the chance for infection. It could take as long as 10-days for skin to heal after a cupping session.

Cupping that is wet can cause small amounts of discomfort as a result of the cuts on the skin. The cuts are not severe and typically heal quickly with no signs of scarring. If the patient is in need of patient, healers can offer the option of administering an local anesthesia to ease the pain.

Needle cupping can be described as a variant of wet cupping where the therapist inserts acupuncture needles, and then place the cups on the body, right over the over the tops of needles. In Chinese practice, needle cupping can assist in the relief of respiratory illnesses, such as the typical cold and bronchitis, and other chest infections as well as pneumonia.

Other kinds of cupping therapy

1. The treatments for cellulite make use of pressure to eliminate out toxins in the body. This helps to promote lymphatic drainage,

boosting circulation, and eliminating adhesions and connective tissue.

2. The spa cupping treatment is used to increase the absorption of treatments applied on the skin, and also to aid in the drainage of stagnant fluids within the body. Spa cupping treatments often include the application of essential oils to boost the therapeutic benefits.

3. The facial cupping process uses small cups and a gentle pressure to raise facial tissues and mimic the movements of lymphatic drainage. Cupping for facial rejuvenation increases circulation and supply of nutrients in the skin cells. This helps soften the appearance of scar tissue, lessen wrinkles and lines on the face decrease muscle tension and tightness, as well as provide relief from the effects of inflammation.

4. The pedi-cupping method combines bio-magnetic reflexology, massage and plantar fascial release massage where specially designed tiny cups are applied to the foot's lower compartment. It's combined with reflexology to relieve of foot pain as well as to boost the healing effects of reflexology.

Chapter 14: History Of Cupping

The exact origins the cupping practice as a treatment method isn't certain. It is however known as an ancient method of treatment which has been employed to cure ailments across a range of cultures. There are ancient accounts in medical textbooks going to thousands of years ago. People who moved between location to another would then carry the practice when they moved to new areas. Alongside its therapeutic purposes it was also employed to remove negative spirits from the patients' bodies and to restore the natural internal equilibrium.

Cupping is most likely to be best known because of its usage in traditional Chinese medicine, but it was practiced by other cultures around the globe and utilized to treat a variety of illnesses. The first types of cupping utilized natural materials like bones, animal horns, and bamboo. Bamboo and animal horns are still used locally in regions like the modern Greece, China, and Vietnam. But, the main part, cupping has evolved away from the use of these natural substances to the more heat-resistant ones like ceramic, silicone or glass cups.

The first recorded reports of cupping were written from the time of the ancient Egyptians, Arabs, Chinese as well as Greeks. Cupping's use in the past was also recorded within Eastern European countries including Russia and the Balkans and Bulgaria as well as in North African as well as Native American cultures.

In many cultures , women were, and continue to be the healers in the community, and consequently, was the one who performed cupping treatments , and handed down their knowledge to the next generation. The majority of people traveled for far distances, often for many days to receive cupping treatments from well-known healers. Unfortunately, many civilizations did not allow women to pursue formal education and, as a result, the majority of their knowledge and their historical records have been lost through time.

Ancient Greeks along with Egyptians

The old Egyptian Hieroglyphic texts Ebers Papyrus, written in about 1500 B.C., is one of the oldest medical texts available around the globe. The hieroglyphic content revealed cupping as a method of treating issues like menstrual irregularities and fever, as well as weakened appetite as well as pain. It also accelerated the healing of illnesses.

There is also evidence to suggest that cupping was utilized for medical purposes in the time of the ancient Greeks. Hippocrates of Kos is known as a Greek physician , also known as the father of Modern Medicine, was born about 400 B.C. Hippocrates is believed to have utilized cupping as a treatment for internal diseases. Another well-known Greek historian and doctor, Herodotus, wrote the following regarding cupping during 413 B.C. :

"Scarification using cupping has the ability to flush out the irritant from the head, of reducing pain from the same region as well as reducing inflammation. of restoring appetite of strengthening stomachs that are weak in removing vertigo as well as fainting and of drawing the deep-seated offending matter toward the surface of drying out the fluids; preventing hemorrhages; stimulating menstrual discharges; stopping the tendency to putrefaction that occurs in fevers, easing rigors, speeding up and slowing down the onset of illness; eliminating the tendency to sleepiness and calming natural rest;

eliminating any heaviness. The above, as well as a myriad of other illnesses, are alleviated by the careful application of cucurbits (cups) either bloody or dry."

Turkish, Arabic, and Persian Cultures

Since to the Greeks and Romans Cupping was an art that cupping was passed down to Turkish, Arabic, and Persian culture. Galen of Pergamon was an Turkish physician surgeon, philosopher, and philosopher who lived between 130 and 200 A.D was a staunch advocate for cupping and was known to suggest it as a remedy for different diseases. Indeed, Galen even went to the point of criticizing of an older Egyptian doctor, Erasistratus who was from Alexandria, who was not a practitioner of cupping.

Wet cupping, sometimes referred to as hijama is a type of medical bleeding that is believed to have been used by early Muslim Arabs and Persians. Hijama can be described as an Arabic word that means "to squeeze" as well as "return to the normal level" of internal equilibrium. The Prophet Mohammed was a prophet who lived between 632 to 570 A.D., was a passionate advocate for wet cupping. He also supported the use of hijama for an act

151

of worship and as a means of treating illnesses, both spiritual and physical. In the period of his time the hijama practice was considered to be the "best of all medicines" as well as highly advised by Muhammad. Actually, hijama has been specifically mentioned in the Quran because of its numerous health benefits.

Other notable historical Arabic doctors who had a hijama practice includes Al- Razi, who lived from 865 until the year 925 A.D., and Ibn Sina -- also referred to as Avicenna - who lived between 980 and 1037 A.D. Since then, Muslim physicians have continued to encourage and improve different cupping methods. Cupping remains a favorite across several Muslim regions of the world and is an essential component of the traditional Perso-Arabic medicine, also referred to in the form of Unani and Yunani Medicine.

Traditional Chinese Medicine

Cupping is among the oldest healing techniques that is used for tradition-based Chinese healing. The Chinese have conducted extensive research regarding the efficacy and benefits from cupping. Much of which was funded by government grants. And it remains a vital element of Chinese medical practice today.

Chinese practitioners typically utilize cupping along with other more well-known types of traditional Chinese treatment, such as Acupressure and acupuncture. In a way, Chinese see cupping as an extension of these methods because it concentrates treatment on the same nerve meridians as well as pressure points that are found throughout the body.

The majority of people who use cupping remain those practicing the traditional Chinese medicine, however it is also utilized by modern Chinese hospitals, and has been modified for various applications, such as the use of chiropractic and massage. Modern Chinese doctors are reported to employ cupping during surgery as a method to redirect bleeding away from the area of surgery.

The earliest accounts suggest that cupping was commonly performed on the members of the early Chinese Imperial Courts as well as other high-ranking individuals. The first records that document cupping's use date to around three thousand years earlier (980

B.C)., when it was said to have been employed as a cure for the pulmonary tuberculosis. Later versions include those of the famous Taoist Ge Hong who lived between 281 and 341 A.D. Ge Hong was well-known for his alchemical practices as well as herbal remedies. He also explained cupping techniques in his book A Handbook of Prescriptions in Emergencies. In the book, he explains the practice of cupping using animal horns to aid in to drain the pus from wounds. This technique was later called jiaofa which is also known as the technique of horns.

Cupping therapy was extensively used in the Tang dynasty (circa 618 to 907 A.D.) in combination with other traditional Chinese treatments for healing like acupuncture and moxibustion. Cupping therapy is used for headaches, dizziness and abdominal pains was described in the ancient texts The Necessities for a Frontier Official that also date in the Tang dynasty. This text offers a comprehensive review of the usage of jiaofa to treat pulmonary tuberculosis as well as related illnesses.

The Supplement to the Outline of Materia Medica, written by Zao Xuemin in the Qing

Dynasty, provides another written description of the use for cupping as a part of tradition Chinese medicine. This book is a part of the Qing Dynasty lasted from 1644 until 1912, and was the final imperial dynasty in China. The book includes an entire chapter on cupping therapies, also called huoquan qi (fire jar Qi). The author provides instructions on how to practice the practice of huoquan Qi by boiling cups made from bamboo or pottery in a solution that has been soaked in herbs before placing them onto the body.

Huoquan Qi is a variant of wet cupping that is like that of the Islamic practices of the hijama that involved piercing the skin using needles used for acupuncture to drain some blood from the area being treated. Huoquan qi was utilized to treat knotted nerves, sore muscles abdominal cramps, joint pain as well as the common cold. It it was also used as a way to treat conditions like rheumatism that would flare in the cold, humid winter seasons.

Cupping is a major part of East Asian countries

Animal horns and other ancient cupping instruments were discovered within Japan, Vietnam, the Korean peninsula, as well as in regions which border China. The findings suggest that cupping was initially invented in China and then spread to other regions due to travel between countries. In Vietnam Cupping was a mix of methods like cupping in water, using air pumps, acupuncture cupping, as well as fire cupping.

European Countries

European physicians have utilized cupping to treat common ailments like the common cold , congestion and chest infections. There are many historical records on the practice of cupping within European cultures , such as those of the Balkans, Bulgaria, Russia and Greece.

Paracelsus, a renowned Swiss medical doctor, alchemist and physician who lived between 1493 and 1541 A.D. is widely regarded as one of the most influential medical researchers in early modern Europe. The famous print, Opus Chyrurgicum, which dates to 1565, shows Paracelsus applying cupping therapies. In the print, a man three women as well as two children in a sauna, their feet immersed in water tubs while the practitioner, likely Paracelsus uses small cups to different parts on their body.

Ambroise Pare was an French barber doctor who lived between 1510 and 1590. She served as the Royal Physician to the Kings Henry II, Francis II, Charles IX, and Henry III. Pare is thought to be one of the pioneers of surgery as well as modern pathology in forensics. She was an early leader in the field of battlefield medicine as well as the treatment of injuries. Like many of his peers, Pare was a proponent of bloodletting and utilized cupping to achieve this treatment. He recommended cupping of the stomach to treat flatulence, and on the abdomen, near the lower rib cage to treat liver and spleen as well as nose bleeding, and even suggested cupping the nipples in order to relieve lung inflammation. However, his most favored cup placement appears to have been placed on the shoulder and neck, which could be used to treat various ailments. A 1649 diagram of the historical period shows three points in the back and the shoulder that are known by the name of Pare Points.

Charles Kennedy was a British surgeon who lived in the first half of the 19th century and was the Physician Extraordinary to The King as well as Director General for the Army Medical Board. The paper he wrote, titled The Essay on Cupping, Etc., Etc., was published in 1826. The paper provided detailed explanations of the methods and equipment used to perform cupping and bloodletting. It also included an extensive examination of numerous ailments which could be treated with cupping or bloodletting.

Cupping as well as Native Americans

Native American healers are known to have utilized a variety of healing techniques, which could be termed alternative medicine in the present. They Native Americans did not have an official written language, as we define it, and there aren't any writings that document exactly when the practice began or the length of time it was practiced. We do know that several tribes used a type of wet cupping. It was used to draw blood from the patient to get rid of bad blood. There isn't any archaeological evidence to establish its origins however, as the instruments are widely used throughout Native Americans cultures, it is possible that cupping originated within North America independently of the different forms of wet cupping like the Islamic hijama, which was popular in other continents.

The equipment utilized to heal Native American healers included a sharp instrument to make the cut and a washed out horn piece or another material to make the cup. Animal horns, like cow horns as well as those from American Bison and Pronghorn Antelope were the most commonly used material used for cupping vessels. However, some tribes utilized hollowed out gourds, bones, or seashells. The vessel was traditionally altered through drilling holes through the narrow part where the healer would apply suction through their mouth.

A lot of Native American healers were women who relied on cupping as a remedy for physical conditions. Cupping doesn't appear to have been seen in the eyes of Native American healers as a magical procedure (i.e. it was not utilized to get rid of evil spirits) however, it was utilized to treat conditions such as headaches dizziness, headaches swelling, rheumatism or blood poisoning. Cupping was generally restricted only to head or the limbs. To treat headaches, a doctor would cut a small cut in the temple of the patient near the vein. The doctor would then put the big part of the horn on the cut and suction the smaller end to draw out the blood. It was then gathered in the dish. In case of blood poisoning, the person was then bled till "all black blood had been drained gone and the blood was clear as well as clear." When the procedure was completed, the doctor would then wrap the cut with astringent to stop bleeding and may apply a natural salve to speed up healing. In certain instances, the treatments were repeated over a period of time until a treatment was considered by the doctor to have been complete.

Chapter 15: What Is Cupping Work?

As we age, our bodies begin to degrade. There is less muscle mass and experience a decline of blood flowing to the adhesions and fascia (connective tissue). This means that the muscle tone diminishes and we become stiffer and wrinkles begin to show. In time, this could result in soreness which makes us are less active, which leads to a further decline in the muscle's tone and blood flow. If we don't take care, this could turn into an endless cycle which results in lower physical activity, which can lead to a diminution in circulation, and so on.

The fundamental idea of the cupping process is to use one of vessels that are open such as glass or silicone bulb or cup is placed on the affected region. Then, a vacuum is formed within the cup. This is accomplished through heating the vessel, then let it cool on the body, or with the help of a tiny pump connected in the container.

"Fire cupping" or "fire cupping" is often utilized to refer to the method where a flame is utilized to heat the interior of the cup to create the vacuum. Typically, this is done by using a candle or similar object that has been

161

which is soaked in rubbing alcohol, and then putting it in the cup to warm it up. Once the fire is taken out after ensuring it's not too hot that it burns the skin the cup is placed over the skin within the area of treatment. The cup will cool as the air inside is dilated, and as it is pressed against the skin, a vacuum is formed. If the suction is too strong, the person who is treating it can alter it by pressing the skin at the edge of the cup, allowing some air into. Additionally, the majority of cups found in modern treatment facilities are equipped with hand-operated valves which permit for the application of suction mechanically through a small hand pump or via tubing to connect to an electric vacuum pump. Glass clear cups are advantageous because they permit the therapist to see the entire process during the treatment.

In all cases it will result in an increase in pressure inside the cup. This pressure is negative and draws the skin upwards to the lip of the cup. This draws blood to the skin's surface and increases blood flow to the muscle beneath as well as connective tissues. The theory is that the negative pressure draws stagnant blood from the region and draws freshly-drawn blood towards the locations in need of healing. This causes an immune response that is mild, that is anti-inflammatory and encourages healing and growth within the affected tissue.

Traditional Chinese medical practices believe that the human body has 12 meridians that have many junctions and nodes along each meridians. These meridians and nodes symbolize the life-force flow lines energy -- qi , or chi -- that circulate through the body. The manipulation or pressure of these points are a good way in order to restore equilibrium to disturbances in the circulation of life energy. Traditional Chinese medical practices teach that it is stagnation of qi and subsequent loss of lymphatic and blood circulation that is the root reason for pain and illness. According to this view the correcting of this imbalance eliminates the blocks in the energy pathways of nature which allows the body to recover itself. Cupping improves local circulation of blood and qi within the region being treated to ease pain, swelling and tension. By drawing impurities towards the skin, it helps to eliminate the toxins.

There are some distinctions among the traditional Chinese practitioners as well as

Western practitioners when it comes to their approach to cupping. Traditional Chinese healers typically view cupping like an expansion of acupuncture or acupressure. using the cups in the same nerve points as well as meridian lines to eliminate obstacles in the body's energy pathways and restore the flow of the qi. They may also offer cupping as part an overall health assessment and may also include recommendations on nutrition, as well as other health-related measures in addition to one-time treatment.

The negative pressure inside the cup pulls the blood from the tissue beneath towards the skin's surface and causes the distinctive black and blue discoloration of the skin around the area being treated. While it might appear like a bruise but it's rarely painful. There isn't a hard or fast rule, however it appears to occur more often in those who are over 40. The discoloration tends to diminish after a series of treatments. The marks usually disappear after just a few days, much like an ordinary bruise.

The treatment is dependent on the type of application. the cups are usually kept on for three to 10 minutes per session. The amount of cups used and their locations in the body will differ based on the type of treatment. The therapist might concentrate on one or more zones of treatment during the session. The cups may remain in one location or, as with massage cupping -- they can be moved slowly across the area of treatment by the therapist, resulting in an effect that is similar to that of deep tissue massage.

It is crucial to ensure that the skin on the area being treated is moisturized prior to beginning the massage procedure. In the event that it is not, the patient could be afflicted by the friction of the skin being drawn into the cup, and then pulled out when the cups move across the area of treatment. It is also essential to ensure that the therapy cup doesn't move across bony parts of the body like shoulders or spinal ridges, since this can cause discomfort for the patient.

A diagram that shows the cupping points of treatment for different illnesses is included in Appendix A near the end of this book.

Chapter 16: Persuasion Of Cupping

Cupping therapy increases blood flow to the area of treatment. This aids in stimulating blood flow and encourage muscular healing. This is why it is now a standard part of the training plans of a variety of top athletes. It has been proven to be an effective technique to treat post-event soreness as well as tired muscles. It is particularly beneficial for athletes participating in sports such as gymnastics, swimming, and track and field because of the constant stress these activities place on muscles and joints. Additionally cupping therapy aids in loosening fascia and breaks down scar tissue. This can dramatically improve the flexibility and range of motion.

It is no doubt that the Olympic gold medalist from America, Michael Phelps, the most accomplished Olympian ever is the most prominent athlete to promote the advantages that cupping therapies offer. In the aftermath of his performance at the 2016 Olympic games in Rio De Janeiro, Brazil TV viewers around the globe were discussing the cupping marks that were clearly visible on his shoulders and back. Then, to get all those awards ... at be honest it was arousing interest for people was stirred.

According to Reuters the sales of cupping therapy equipment increased 20% in the weeks after Michael Phelps' performance at the Olympic Games. The International Cupping Therapy Association reported that they witnessed fifty percent more healthcare professionals who sought the certification needed to provide cupping therapy.

Chapter 17: The Benefits Of Cupping

While Cupping has been practiced for centuries but some in the medical profession continue to doubt its effectiveness. The critics of cupping therapy say that the benefits of cupping are psychosomatic which is due to a strong placebo effect. They also claim that it only creates a sense of relaxation, without offering any actual health benefits.

It's possible that it's the case, however it is still to be advocated and used by some of the top athletes around the world. This is quite convincing and supports the use of it as a treatment method to heal physical injuries and also in the treatment of certain diseases.

Michael Phelps and other top-tier athletes are known to use massage cupping and myofascial compression to ease muscle pain to aid in recovering from injuries and improve mobility. This kind of cupping therapy has also been proven that it is effective for releasing muscle connective tissue tightness as well as in removing scar tissue, and in treating knotted muscles and swelling joints. When performed by skilled experts, skilled practitioners, cupping therapy is able to aid sufferers with a myriad of diseases. It has been demonstrated to increase circulation and blood flow to the tissues and muscles which increases the supply for oxygenation to the cells and loosening muscles fibers and knotted nerves and facilitating the draining of lymphatic fluids out of the body.

The practitioners of hijama, Huoquan Qi, and other types of wet cupping believe that suction pulls stagnant or "bad" blood to the area of treatment and that the removal of this blood causes the elimination of toxins as well as other harmful substances that cause discomfort for the human body. The practitioners also advocate the benefits of wet cupping as a method of preventing or treating certain diseases like headaches, colds and flu as well as respiratory ailments like bronchitis, or pneumonia.

Since wet cupping involves the making of tiny cuts, punctures or abrasions to face, the skin is at risk. There is a chance of getting infected. Therefore, wet cupping is best done under safe, clean conditions. The majority of patients won't feel any major discomfort, however if you are experiencing discomfort, you should inquire of your therapists for the local anesthetic for the area to reduce the sensitization of the area as cupping is meant to be a therapeutic experience and not a painful one. When the cupping session is over the therapist must cleanse the area to eliminate any blood. They should then apply antiseptic to the affected area and cover it with suitable bandaging. The area must be kept dry and clean just like with any other wound to facilitate speedy healing and lessen the chance for infection.

In some cases practitioners can combine cupping and the acupuncture. In such cases, needles used for acupuncture are initially placed into the skin, and then the cups are placed on top of the needles. Like acupuncture and Acupressure therapy, this technique is utilized to repair problems with the flow of Qi in the body and is typically coupled with or followed by a deep massage of the tissues. Therapists can also carry out the hydration of the area to decrease the amount of bruising or discoloration.

Cupping Therapy to Detoxification

Since the beginning it has been utilized to eliminate stagnant blood and eliminating harmful compounds from your body. Cupping has been used over the centuries to treat a variety of circulatory and blood conditions, including hemophilia, anemia and high blood pressure as well as varicose veins. It has also been effective in treating numerous ailments not related to the circulatory system. These include arthritis and rheumatic conditions including gout, infertility, and other gynecological issues depression, migraines, anxiety and asthma. and skin disorders like eczema, psoriasis and acne.

In the view of the theorists the theory, the pressure that is created by suction in the cups pulls the blood stagnant and toxins up to the capillaries at the skin's surface so that they can be removed out of the body. After the toxins are eliminated, the body is liberated to begin healing itself. In addition patients often experience the increase of energy after treatment.

Alongside alleviating pain, this study demonstrated the statistically important improvement in raising the temperatures of skin (an indicator of increased the circulation of blood) and lower blood pressure. It was concluded by the study that cupping can provide the potential to help in managing nerve and joint pain , as and relief from respiratory problems like coughing and breathing difficulties.

A study conducted in 2012 showed that cupping therapy was able to provide substantial relief of knee and neck pain. Some patients reported that treatment was efficient for up to 12 weeks after treatment. Additionally, those who had received cupping treatments also reported an improvement in their overall feeling of wellbeing and improved pressure thresholds than those who had massage therapy with no cupping.

Chapter 18: What To Expect From Cupping

Before any therapy session with cupping the patient must discuss any concerns regarding the treatment with their practitioner and explain the reason why they're receiving the cupping treatment. The therapist will inquire about the kind of discomfort or pain you are feeling, as well as the location in the body, to ensure they place cupping cups on the most effective locations to treat.

The exact number and location and position of your cups along with the length of the treatment is determined by your therapist , based on the condition being addressed. The back, however, is the most frequently that is used for cupping therapy due to the abundance of nerves that run through the spine and back, and due to the fact that the back has five meridian lines along which to place the therapy.

If the cups are applied onto the skin patients may feel sensation of a tightness or pull from the skin that is being pulled to the. Each person is unique If you feel this feeling painful, tell your doctor so that they can modify the procedure to suit the specific needs of your.

Although cupping can cause visible swelling and bruising on the site It is a generally painful. The marks that occur after the cupping treatment can be present for a couple of days to several weeks and should not leave any lasting marks. The bruises themselves are the result of ruptures of the capillaries as blood is drawn towards the skin's surface. Although they appear they shouldn't cause pain however there could be some irritation when the body cleanses itself of blood cells that remain which are the cause of the discoloration. In rare instances there is a possibility that the patient will get a skin infection however, when they do happen they are usually rather small.

Cupping with water is not recommended without a prior medical assessment by a doctor for those who suffer from hemophilia or any other bleeding disorders, or who are taking anticoagulants. Cupping therapy is also not recommended for those who suffer from inflammation, irritation or burns that affect the skin. Conditions that require discussion with your physician prior getting cupping therapy. These include:

* Hemophilia and other bleeding disorders

* A pregnancy that is suspected or known.

* Possible or confirmed bone fractures

* Active muscles spasms

* Diabetic ulcers

* Deep Vein Thrombosis

* Skin cancers and metastatic cancers that have taken over one part within the body

Cupping isn't typically done on the forehead or the head. If you suffer from headaches it is generally done on muscles or nerves of the neck, shoulder and back muscles. but not using cups on the forehead or temples.

Do you want to try cupping? If you're an avid athlete or who is extremely demanding for their body, and is trying to find a way to alleviate your pains and aches I think it's worth taking into consideration. In addition to those looking for alternative methods of treatment that are not offered by the standard western healthcare institutions Cupping is an option that should be considered. Evidence suggests its efficacy, but the degree of benefits will differ depending on the patient. If you're suffering, try the cupping a shot before you write it off. Research and evidence from anecdotal sources suggest that cupping could be an effective addition to other methods for managing pain. There isn't any evidence of any negative side consequences, so other than the expense of treatment and the possibility of having visible marks for few days the risk is minimal.

As evident in the widely-reported images from Michael Phelps from the 2016 Olympics Some skin discoloration is anticipated, especially if the treatment is applied to the chest, back, or shoulder regions on the human body. It usually appears as circular marks that match the size of the cups that begin red, before becoming into a darker shade of swollen skin. Although they can look a bit scary but they are more painful than they actually feel.

The typical deep dark spots of discoloration in the area of treatment typically will last for several weeks, however in rare cases, it can last up to two weeks. Like bruising caused by an injury The discoloration is the result of ruptures in capillaries resulting from the blood flowing up onto the face's surface. Some cupping professionals believe that the amount of discoloration can be a sign of the quantity of toxins within the body of a patient and areas with high levels of toxins leaving prominent signs. In line with this, people who have less discoloration on the skin are believed to have less contaminants in the body. Most of the time, the coloration diminishes after repetition of sessions. This indicates that the cupping is working in removing the stagnant blood and toxins out of the area being treated. Making sure that the body is properly hydrated prior to any cupping treatment, and following that with a gentle massage on the area of treatment can lessen the swelling and discoloration that is experienced in the patients.

Other adverse effects of the cupping could include discomfort, irritation or burning sensation. There could be the possibility of developing a skin infection. It is recommended that the patient consult with a medical professional or a practitioner who practices traditional Chinese medicine regarding the possible benefits and potential negative side effects prior to starting treatment which involves cupping as a stand-alone treatment or as a part of other methods of treatment. Patients may also be afflicted with lightheadedness or feel warm sensations accompanied by sweating when they undergo treatment. If you notice these signs be sure to inform your therapist they can alter the treatment so that you can rest and recuperate before heading home.

It is also important to note that in the event that the procedure is done by a child, the bruises and discolorations after cupping can be misinterpreted as evidence of abuse in a child. So, should you observe someone looking at the marks with suspicion or squinting, it's best to let them know to avoid any confusion.

In the end, the low risk of adverse side effects in conjunction with the potential advantages can be a strong argument for the treatment of cupping.

Chapter 19: How To Locate The Cupping

Practitioner And What Is The Cost To Receive

Cupping Therapy

Cupping therapy is provided by a range of professionals that include those who practice traditional Chinese therapy massage therapists, acupuncturists as well as physiotherapists, sports medical experts nurses, medical professionals chiropractors, as well as other practitioners of healing arts.

To find a practitioner search for a clinic that has been recognized by an national or state-based accrediting body such as the State or National Acupuncture Board or the National Certification Commission for Acupuncture and Oriental Medicine (NCCAOM). Practitioners who are certified by these organizations are required to complete more than 3,000 hours of instruction at a recognized school and pass a series of necessary tests in order to ensure that they are able to offer the safest and legally-approved practice of acupuncture as well as cupping therapy.

A total cupping session may be anywhere between 15 and 60 minutes. A one-hour session is typically consist of 15 to 20 minutes of massage, five minutes to apply the cups for 15 to 20 minutes with the cups firmly on the skin. Then another 5 minutes for the removal of the cups as well as 15-20 minutes for massage after the session.

Consult your physician before you begin cupping or other alternative or complementary therapy. Also, talk with your cupping practitioner, also, prior to trying the practice. Here are some questions you could ask your cupping therapist:

* What are the conditions they recommend cupping?

What are their qualifications?

* What are their experiences with cupping? And for whatpurpose?

What are the treatment options I am given the same as the treatments that are standard for my particular condition?

What are the side effects been reported in other patients? Are there any reasons why I shouldn't take cupping?

Cupping therapy is an effective and safe method for non-invasive treatment, it's always recommended to seek out an experienced therapist prior to seeking treatment. It is also essential to verify qualifications of the therapist prior to getting treatment. Check to see if the therapy provider has the necessary credentials to practice cupping, and also provide you with all the specifics of the process. It is best to choose an expert who can answer all of your concerns. To ensure that you feel at ease you can ask for testimonials from former patients prior to undergoing treatment.

Who Shouldn't Do Cupping?

Cupping is safe for people who are in good health overall. However, as a preventative option, some therapists decide not to do cupping for certain patients, like pregnant women or hemophiliacs, who are vulnerable to bleeding excessively. In addition, patients experiencing convulsions, fever or cramps shouldn't be treated with cupping and instead get medical attention by a doctor. It is also essential to ensure that the doctor takes care to inspect the skin around the area of treatment for indications of ulcers or open wounds, that could result in infection.

People suffering from severe allergies are also not usually suggested to have cupping. Menstruating or pregnant women as well as patients with metastatic cancer or fractures are not permitted to undergo to undergo the treatment. Additionally, patients who are taking blood thinners or suffer from conditions that block blood clotting may be advised against cupping. A therapist who has had the appropriate training can examine patients with care and assist them decide if cupping is suitable for the patient's particular situation.

Conclusion

Cupping for sports is a new technique that blends traditional methods of cupping alongside the latest concepts of physical therapy. Presently, a variety of physical therapy clinics are slowly adapting the practice of cupping athletes to aid in increasing recuperation and alleviating post-workout pain. To maximize the benefits of this technique during sports, experts have the expertise to help you. For those who prefer to perform these exercises at home at your own pace, they could be extremely efficient in relieving muscle pain. It is best to work with a friend while doing this at home.

I hope this book can assist you gain further information on cupping for sports and its many advantages. If you decide to do your cupping at home , or obtain a professional certification cupping is an intriguing subject to master and a breeze to master when you have the proper understanding.

www.ingramcontent.com/pod-product-compliance
Lightning Source LLC
Chambersburg PA
CBHW062116040426
42336CB00041B/1240